A Lifetime with Hopkins

A Lifetime with Hopkins

Peter Milward, S.J.

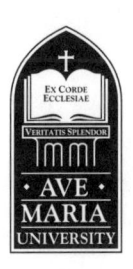

Sapientia Press
of Ave Maria University

Copyright © 2005 by Sapientia Press of Ave Maria University, Naples, Florida. All rights reserved.

No part of this publication may be reproduced or transmitted in any form or means, electronic or mechanical, including photography, recording, or any other information storage or retrieval system, without permission in writing from the publisher.

Requests for permission to make copies of any part of the work should be directed to:

Sapientia Press
of Ave Maria University
24 Frank Lloyd Wright Drive
Ann Arbor, MI 48106
888-343-8607

Cover Design: Eloise Anagnost

Printed in the United States of America

Library of Congress Control Number: 2005900805

ISBN 1-932589-22-8

Table of Contents

Preface vii

Hopkins and I 1
The Piedness of Beauty 5
This World of Wales 9
Shock in Hopkins 15
The Echo Principle in Hopkins 19
The Two Vocations 25
The Poems of 1879 33
"Spring and Fall", 1980 37
The Worst of Hopkins 43
Hopkins's "Comfort" 49
Hopkinsian Reminiscences 55
The Circling Bird 65
The Place of Hopkins in Poetic Tradition 73
The Message of Hopkins 79
Hopkins and the Oxford Movement 89

Table of Contents

Hopkins and the Spirit of Man 99

Hopkins as Ecological Prophet 105

This-ness in Hopkins 111

Hopkins and the Renaissance of Rhythm 119

"The Dearest Freshness" 131

Hamlet in Hopkins 137

Twin Beacons in the Life of Hopkins 145

Hopkins and the Imagery of Procreation 155

Hopkins's Commentary on Newman's *Grammar* 163

Finding God in Hopkins 171

The Self as Other in Hopkins 179

The Eccentricity of Hopkins 189

Hopkins in Ireland 197

Index 209

Preface

Here is a selection of essays that I have contributed over the years to *Hopkins Research*, the annual publication of the Hopkins Society of Japan from the time of its first issue in 1972. As honorary president of the society from its inception, I have felt an obligation, or rather an inner compulsion, to contribute an article to each succeeding issue; and as the years have passed, I find I have amassed a considerable number of such articles—which from my English and Jesuit education I prefer to call "essays". In putting them together, I have avoided arranging them in categories, which might appear arbitrary and forced, but I have preferred to follow the line of least resistance and leave them in their original chronological order, as they have appeared year by year from the beginning till the present—with a few gaps, where an essay had already been published elsewhere.

As for the title imposed on this miscellaneous collection, *A Lifetime with Hopkins*, it is sufficiently explained by one of the following essays entitled "Hopkinsian Reminiscences". For my association with the poet goes back, willy-nilly, to my very birth as a Londoner and my baptism as a Catholic.

Lastly, I wish to make acknowledgments in this Preface not only to the Hopkins Society of Japan, under whose aegis I have produced so many articles on the poet, but also to the organizers of the Hopkins International Summer School at Monasterevin in Ireland, for which I have presented not a few of those articles in a setting surprisingly congenial to Hopkins himself, despite his sad experiences in Dublin during the last five years of his life. For this we both, "Hopkins and I", have to thank the prime mover, the Irish poet, Desmond Egan.

—Peter Milward, SJ

Hopkins and I

THE TITLE of this chapter may seem somewhat egocentric, but it refers to something very deep both in the poetry of Hopkins and in the reader's response. In the style of Newman's motto, *"Cor ad cor loquitur"*—Heart speaks to heart—Hopkins might well have added to his own line "Myself it speaks and spells" the completing phrase "to another self". After all, there is no true speech in an empty solitude.

Hopkins is indeed the most personal of poets, both in himself and to others. In his religious poetry he expresses a personal relationship between himself and God, as in his famous opening line of "The Wreck of the Deutschland", "*Thou* mastering *me*"—where he seems to echo the deep conviction of his spiritual guide Newman on "two luminous beings". Thus he is at once egocentric and theocentric, with the one quality deeply rooted in the other.

In his view of nature, moreover, Hopkins discerns selfhood present in all things, as the peculiar quality of "thisness" bespeaking a native splendour in them. Everywhere in the natural world, he exclaims, "self flashes off frame and face". But most of all it does so in moments of intense stress, as when in "The Windhover", he says, "I caught this morning morning's minion . . . in his riding". In such moments the poet's "heart in hiding" is filled with rapture, impelling him to praise God, whom he sees present in all that beauty.

Further, in his theory of poetry it is Hopkins's aim as a poet to arrest what he sees in the natural world, to express his perception in apt words, and to convey the same impression to his readers. Only, because words in Victorian English have become so lamentably dull and conventionalised, he feels the necessity of renewing them in their original strength, of altering their syntactical structure, and of reforming them in unaccustomed compounds, while compacting them in a new "sprung rhythm"—and all to lay fresh emphasis on the stress of divine mystery in the world of nature.

Thus, running through the poetry of Hopkins, there is an almost bewildering series of selves merging into each other. First, there is the divine Self, which is manifested in all phenomena of nature, especially in their pied and dappled variety. Secondly, there are the separate selves of natural things, which flash out most vividly in times of stress. Thirdly, there is the hidden self of the poet, which is elicited by his perception of the selfhood in and behind all things, and which is exercised by his endeavour to give apt expression to it. Fourthly, there is the self of the reader, to whom the poetry is addressed.

In other words, implied in this theory of poetry is a deep metaphysical perception that self is not only (in scholastic terms) a principle of individuation but also a principle of communication. It is not only what every being has most proper and native to himself but also what he desires to communicate most deeply to other beings, "crying *What I do is me, for that I came.*"

There is, however, one important modification to be made to this theory of poetry in terms of a paradox: namely, that the communication of self is possible only through the renunciation of self. True selfhood requires an infinite giving of self to others, a perpetual going out from one's self to others. This is the fundamental meaning of the climax to "The Windhover", by which beings have to "fall, gall themselves, and gash gold-vermilion". Or as the poet puts it in the opening stanza of "The Wreck", one has to become "almost unmade" in order to feel the fresh touch of God's finger.

This modification is what Hopkins not only uttered but also experienced in the course of his poetic life—from the time he renounced his poetry on entering the Society of Jesus, by way of the first breaking of his "elected silence" to compose "The Wreck", to his culminating experience of the divine darkness recorded in his "terrible sonnets". Through all these stages there was formed within the hidden recess of his selfhood what he hails in one of his greatest poems as "immortal diamond".

Then, through the poems a similar process is gradually signified and effected in the mind and self of the reader, as by constant rereading and reflection they become part of his selfhood.

(*Hopkins Research* 1, March 1972)

The Piedness of Beauty

WHAT IS BEAUTY? "The splendour of order," answers the philosopher. The ordered relation of parts to each other and to the whole produces on the human mind an impression of splendour and radiance. But this order needn't be perfectly geometrical or symmetrical, as the orthodoxy of the Renaissance required. That is only one kind of order—classical, artificial order. But there is another kind of order, more natural, less attached to symmetry, one that "snatches a grace beyond the reach of art". Such was the order, such the beauty, admired by Hopkins.

The beauty Hopkins celebrates in his poems is a wild, barbarous, uncultivated beauty, the beauty rather of lakes and mountains than of gardens and meadows. He feels paradoxically more at home where there is less homeliness or domesticity—in the North rather than the South, in the West rather than the East. He delights in the "brute beauty" of the windhover, as he rings "upon the rein of a wimpling wing in his ecstasy", or of the uncaged skylark, unfettered amid "his free fells". He delights, too, in the "beauty bright" of men, whether in mould or in mind, their "beauty and valour and act", which are both for themselves and for him motives of pride and of blessing.

More precisely, what he finds most to his taste in all this "brute beauty" is its endless variety, in which every whole is composed of parts that are each unique in its own way, so that at every level of existence, from the tiniest grain or drop to the vast immensity of the universe, the uniqueness of the *haecceitas*, or this-ness, of things reigns supreme. For this purpose he uses many words in his own characteristic sense. His favourite word is doubtless "dappled" as an adjective, "dapple" as a noun and verb. "Glory be to God for dappled things" is one of his best-known lines. He thinks of sunrise as "dapple dawn" and of sunset as "dappled with damson". He rejoices in the varied colour of apple blossom in the orchard as "drop-of-blood-and-foam-dapple".

This is what Hopkins means by the "piedness" of beauty. It isn't just the plain contrast of black and white in magpies or piebald ponies, but a more varied contrast, such as he details in the six-line octet of "Pied Beauty", beginning with "skies of couple-colour" (where he is presumably thinking of "the jay-blue heavens of pied and peeled May"). For him "pied" has evidently more of blue in its notion than of black, as when he later speaks of skies that "betweenpie mountains" with an azure smile.

All this is, however, merely "mortal beauty". That is to say, it all looks beyond the parti-coloured contrasts of earthly hues in the daytime to the stark contrast between life and death, day and night, light and darkness. Here is also the fundamental movement of Hopkins's mind in his sonnets taken as a whole. They may all be seen as together passing from the brightness of day to the darkness of night, as he describes it most vividly in "Spelt from Sibyl's Leaves". Then it is that earth's "dapple is at an end", and the uniqueness of earthly things is no longer apparent to the senses. But then he comes to realize all the more vividly the essential vividness of "black, white; right, wrong", as earth appears in stark contrast to heaven, as though in a final apocalypse, which is literally an "uncovering" or "revealing".

The mortal beauty of the day may serve for a time to "keep warm men's wits to the things that are". But it is also dangerous in the way it captivates men's wits and leads them astray along the path to death. At best, it provides a pointer to and a reminder of another beauty that is "past change", or in plain terms, "God's better beauty, grace". In him the beauty of changing things is retained unchanged in youthful loveliness and innocence. In his infinitely rich simplicity is to be found in perfect form the rich variety of things. To him all must be resigned in time, that it may be retained in eternity. Thus for Hopkins the poetic contemplation of creatures inevitably leads his mind to adoration of the Creator in a universal and unending prayer.

(*Hopkins Research* 2, March 1973)

This World of Wales

"LOVE" IS A WORD which, with all its variants, deeply appeals to the heart of Hopkins. In "The Wreck of the Deutschland" he speaks of "the loveable west", which he identifies as "a pastoral forehead of Wales". And in his subsequent sonnet "In the Valley of the Elwy" he expands on the loveliness of his home at St. Beuno's. It is filled with inscapes of nature, trees and rivers, hills and valleys, "landscape plotted and pieced". It seems ideally suited to the composition of such poems as he excelled in. And in fact it inspired him to compose the series of his happiest poems, the "bright sonnets".

Above and around the particular inscapes of nature Hopkins relishes "all the air things wear". This is what he noticed from the first moment of his new life at St. Beuno's College. In a letter to his father, written the day after his arrival, he describes how "the house stands on a steep hillside, it commands the long-drawn valley of the Clwyd to the sea, a vast prospect, and opposite is Snowdon and its range". Then he adds, "The air seems to me very fresh and wholesome."

This was for the poet an important condition of his poetic inspiration, considering the emphasis he laid on the interconnection between the spiritual and the material. The air was for him the element surrounding him as the mother's womb surrounds her child, "this air, which by life's law/ My lung must draw and draw." Amid the hills of Wales he felt it all the more keenly as "wild air, world-mothering air,/ Nestling me everywhere."

It may have been the fact of his living on a hill in Wales (Maenefa, also known as Benarth from the name of a farmhouse situated on its slope) that directed his thoughts to the wide valley spreading out before him every moment of the day. This was not the Valley of the Elwy mentioned in the title of this poem, but the larger Vale of Clwyd through which the river of that name meanders down to the sea beyond the "shallow and frail town" of Rhyl. The Elwy is merely a tributary of the Clwyd, flowing down from the hills through the cathedral city of St. Asaph before entering the larger river.

Now why is this sonnet named after the river Elwy? Is it because the Elwy was a more beautiful river than the sluggish Clwyd? Or was it because the poet was accustomed, as we know from his other sonnet entitled "Hurrahing in Harvest", to go fishing there? Yet we know he had reasons for dissociating this poem, in spite of its title, from any connection with his temporary home at St. Beuno's College. The opening words of the sonnet, "I remember a house where all were good to me," might seem to refer to St. Beuno's, but for the poet's own assurance, in a letter to Bridges, that "the kind people of the sonnet were the Watsons of Shooter's Hill, London, nothing to do with the Elwy". He doesn't even come to the Elwy in the poem till he approaches the sestet; and here he devotes only two lines to a general description of its beauty: "Lovely the woods, waters, meadows, combes, vales,/ All the air things wear that build this world of Wales."

The main theme of the poem, as Hopkins outlines it to Bridges in the same letter, is, in fact, a contrast between the house in Shooter's Hill, "where all were good to me", and "the inmate" of Wales, who "does not correspond" to the loveliness of his country. What he finds in common to the countryside of Kent and Wales is indeed the loveliness of their respective landscapes: but where they differ from each other is the inner disposition of their inhabitants. Within, he expects to find a goodness commensurate with the outer beauty; but that isn't what he finds in Wales or the Welsh. Apparently, somewhere in the Valley of the Elwy Hopkins had had an unpleasant encounter with one or more of the local inhabitants, possibly owing to a prohibition of his fishing, and this may have coloured his whole impression of them.

His notion of loveliness is on the whole expressed more frequently with regard to human beings than inanimate nature. In one poem he speaks of "world's loveliest—men's selves", and in another, more precisely, of "the loveliness of youth". He sees Christ himself playing "in ten thousand places,/ Lovely in limbs and lovely in eyes not his". It is an ideal he finds realized more in children and young boys than in grown men, associated with "innocent mind and Mayday" and "chastity in mansex fine".

On the other hand, the poet is all too often cheated of his ideal in the men he meets in real life. They are still "dear" to him, but all too "dogged" and obstinate. So he comments, in connection with another river, the Ribble in Lancashire, on "the heir to his own selfbent so bound, so tied to his turn". For the most part, he sees man as a rebel, fixed in malice, needing to be mastered by God "with wrecking and storm", and the world he lives in as a "bent world". Thus the Welsh "inmate", living by the banks of the Elwy, is by no means unique in doggedness or malice, but his unkindness stands out all the more in contrast to the loveliness of his surroundings.

This theme is developed, again in a Welsh setting, in the sonnet "The Sea and the Skylark". Here, too, the poet contrasts the loveliness of such natural sounds as the roar of the breaking waves and the song of a skylark with the "shallow and frail town" of Rhyl. Here, too, "the inmate does not correspond" to his surroundings. But here the closing impression is one of sadness, if not sourness. For it is on the latter, less pleasant half of the contrast that the poet ends. Men, he laments, "have lost that cheer and charm of earth's past prime", and they are now declining to "man's last dust", now draining fast "to man's first slime".

There is no such pessimism at the end of "In the Valley of the Elwy". The whole poem is brightened by the opening description of the "house where all were good to me", nor is this impression seriously impaired in the sestet. Indeed, without the poet's own allusion to the Watsons of Shooter's Hill, we would naturally have taken him to refer to some house in the Valley of the Elwy, as suggested by the title, or more generally in "this world of Wales". Even the qualifying line about the "inmate" is less shocking than "this shallow and frail town" in the other poem. Its meaning is in any case rather obscure. Who, we wonder, is "the inmate", and to what does he "not correspond"? And "inmate" is a rather odd word to use for "inhabitant", indicating, as it seems to do, an asylum. What is more important is that the poet doesn't merely leave the "inmate" in the obscurity of his malice, as he leaves the town of Rhyl in its shallowness and frailty. He rather goes on to pray for his completion and well-being. As in the first part of "The Wreck", he turns to the Father with an earnest petition not so much for a "rebel" as for "thy creature dear". For whatever unkindness he may have received from the Welsh, or more precisely from those dwelling in the Valley of the Elwy, he still feels fondness for them. And this fondness he here attributes to the Father.

Then will the loveliness of these "woods, waters, meadows, combes, vales" be all the more deeply appreciated, both by the poet himself and by the Welsh "inmate", when the latter is as he should be. For their natural inscape is not in himself alone, but also in the eye of the beholder. Nor is it enough, though he seems to say so in "Hurrahing in Harvest", for the two once to meet and then "the heart rears wings bold and bolder". Rather, the eye of the beholder has to look beyond the things in themselves to the presence of our Saviour within them and to praise him in them. This is precisely what Hopkins desired for the Welsh around him, and what prompted him soon after his arrival at St. Beuno's "to feel a desire to do something for the conversion of Wales". For then, he felt, the "inmate" would at last correspond to the "charm and instress of Wales", and then he would breathe in what is freshest in its air. For the material cannot long endure without the spiritual, nor the natural without the supernatural, nor "mortal beauty" without "God's better beauty, grace".

(*Hopkins Research* 4, July 1975)

Shock in Hopkins

It is a characteristic theory of Elisabeth Schneider in her book *The Dragon at the Gate* (1968) that the vision of Christ presented in the crucial stanza 28 of "The Wreck of the Deutschland" is no mere poetic imagination of Hopkins or hallucination of the nun in a moment of tension, but an objective supernatural event in which she saw Christ's very self. It is also implied that this event was experienced not only by the nun on that occasion, but also by the poet himself on an analogous occasion.

This theory is quoted with approval by Alison Sulloway in her book on *Gerard Manley Hopkins and the Victorian Temper* (1972), where she further justifies it with reference to "Hopkins's strange letter to Dixon on the nature of miraculous visitations" (Oct. 23, 1886). In this letter Hopkins is speaking apropos of Wordsworth's "Immortality" ode about men who have "seen something" and received a shock which has left them "in a tremble ever since". In his opinion Wordsworth was one such man, and it was when he wrote his great ode that "human nature got another of those shocks" and "the tremble of it is spreading". From these words, says Sulloway, we may conclude that Hopkins had in turn experienced a similar shock in writing his own ode, not just vicariously in the nun, but directly in some personal vision, though, she adds, "the exact nature of his vision was a private matter".

Before going further, I wish to state my substantial agreement with both Schneider and Sulloway. All I intend to propose here is partly a modification, partly an addition to their theory. Both seem to relate Hopkins's vision too closely to that of the nun in stanza 28, though this is surely a poetic imagination based on the gospel incident in Matthew 14. Both seem to overlook the fact that the poet has already indicated the exact nature of his vision in the autobiographical part of his poem in stanza 2: "Thou knowest the walls, altar and hour and night". It is surely the same experience that is recalled in the later sonnet "Carrion Comfort": "That night of now done darkness." In both passages the poet describes his experience in terms not of Christ coming over the waters "in the storm of his strides", as he did to the disciples on Genesareth and to the nun on the North Sea, but of Jacob wrestling with the angel, as described in Genesis 32. On that occasion his impression of Christ was not, at first, one of comfort, but of terror "at lightning and lashed rod", in spite of which he humbly "kissed the rod" and confessed Christ. Then it was that in lightning he found the love, in winter he found the warmth, of God.

There is yet another important implication in this account, which neither Schneider nor Sulloway has noticed. In his letter to Dixon, Hopkins speaks not only of Wordsworth's ode, while no doubt thinking of his own, but also of Blake, recalling the occasion when that poet "fell into hysterical excitement" at his first hearing of the ode. He is here citing Blake as "a proof of the power of the shock", while no doubt thinking of himself as affording another such proof. In his own case, Hopkins not only was a recipient of the shock, but also (like Wordsworth) gave it poetic expression in his ode on "The Wreck". So it isn't perhaps without significance that he describes Blake as "a most poetically electrical subject both active and passive". As a passive subject, Blake had responded to the shock "at his first hearing" of Wordsworth's ode; but when had he been an active subject and given poetic expression to his shock?

The answer to this question is, I submit, to be found in Blake's well-known but little understood poem "The Tyger". What this poem expresses is, above all, a strange supernatural terror, culminating in a question which seems to contradict the innocent affirmation of "The Lamb": "Did he who made the Lamb make thee?" Here is, in my opinion, no mere question of religious doubt, for which Blake himself would have condemned the doubter to mockery in "Age and Death" ("Auguries of Innocence"). Still less is it a rhetorical question expecting the Manichean answer "No". It is rather a question whose answer the poet knows only too well; and this makes him tremble all through his being, so that he can't bring himself to say what Hopkins said, and what Simon Peter had said before them, "I did say Yes."

It is true that Hopkins never refers openly to Blake's poem, but it seems to be strongly implied both in his letter to Dixon and in "The Wreck" itself. It certainly fits in with the strong apocalyptic element in Hopkins's ode, which is rightly emphasized by Sulloway, as arising out of the Oxford Movement and the earlier evangelical morality preached by Wilberforce. For of all English poets Blake was outstandingly influenced by apocalyptic ideas, which contributed not a little to making him, in Hopkins's eyes, "crazy", "unstrung", and "hysterical". He had the shock, but not the theology to interpret it in universal terms. Hopkins, however, was enabled by his study of Catholic theology to interpret the shock both poetically and theologically in terms of "the stress felt" and "the stroke dealt". Here he implicitly identifies Blake's "Tyger" (as T. S. Eliot was later to do explicitly in "Gerontion") with him whom Peter had confessed to be "the Christ, the Son of the living God". In this terrified recognition, moreover, instead of becoming crazy like Blake, Hopkins found only serenity and peace of mind, in "the heart of the Host".

(*Hopkins Research* 5, September 1976)

The Echo Principle in Hopkins

ONE OF HOPKINS'S favourite poems, which has however been less favoured by readers and commentators, is his double poem "The Leaden Echo and the Golden Echo", which he composed for "the maidens' song" in his unfinished drama, "St. Winefred's Well". Commenting on it in a letter to Canon Dixon in 1886, he claimed that he had "never done anything more musical". Part of the music in this poem consists in its frequent use of verbal echoes, especially on the word "beauty" in both parts, then on the word "despair", as constituting the leaden echo, and then on the other word "yonder", as constituting the golden echo. This is all obvious enough, and hardly worth mentioning. But there is one more important echo, if less highly appreciated by critics, which serves as a structural link between the two parts of the poem. It is the echo of the final "despair" at the end of "The Leaden Echo" in "Spare!"—meaning "Wait!" or "Stay!"—at the beginning of "The Golden Echo".

What I wish to point out here is that this echo isn't merely a structural device, still less a cheap trick or tour de force, linking the two parts of the poem together. Rather, it serves to emphasize something in the poetic theory of Hopkins which hasn't been generally noticed by critics, partly because the poet refrained from adverting to it in any explicit way.

For echo in its widest sense is surely fundamental to the whole poetic method of Hopkins. As a poet, he uses words to their fullest extent as well for their musical as for their meaningful qualities, as well for their sound as for their sense. It is his aim, like that of T. S. Eliot after him, to reach through words to an effect of music. And for this purpose he strains his talent to select and arrange words for their resonance. More than any other poet in English literature, since the days of the Old English alliterative verse, he rings the changes on consonants and vowels, so as to make them repeatedly and variedly chime with each other.

Considering the revolutionary nature of Hopkins's prosody and use of language in almost every respect, it is surprising to note that in one respect at least he clings tenaciously to recent poetic tradition. This is in his constant use of rhyme, especially in his sonnets. Whereas he was ready to give up other rules of prosody that had been imported from mediaeval France in the time of Chaucer, he remained faithful to the use of rhyme, though it was already being abandoned by poets in his own time, notably by Walt Whitman. Why? Simply, I would suggest, because rhyme, both end rhyme and internal rhyme, was part and parcel of his echo principle.

To explain this point, let me turn to his poem "Inversnaid", where we find a similar use of echo in connection with "despair". Only, here Despair is spelt with a capital "D" in personified form: "It rounds and rounds Despair to drowning." Here, in addition to the rhyme of "frowning" and "drowning", there is a rhyming repetition of "rounds", connected by assonance with "and", and a significant alliteration of "Despair" with "drowning", while the sound of "r" reverberates throughout the line. It is indeed impressive to note how every word chimes in a complex pattern with every other word, not neglecting the seemingly insignificant words "It" and "to". Everything seems to be conspiring to pull Despair down "to drowning" in the murky depths of the pitchblack pool.

But again, as in "The Leaden Echo", the very depth of despair in the moment of drowning serves to revive hope. Or in the personified terms of the poem, the death of Despair is the resurrection of Hope. So we find it here, in the word "rounds". This appears not so much within the poem itself, as in comparison with the poem which follows it in most editions, "As kingfishers catch fire". In this latter poem we may observe an echo, verbal perhaps, yet (I submit) more than merely verbal, between the verb "rounds" and the adjective "roundy" applied to "wells" into which stones are "tumbled over rim" and "ring".

Here Hopkins passes from the kingfishers and dragonflies of the opening line to the echoing resonance of stones in wells and bells in towers. Between these two similes there is at once a comparison of sound, reinforced by the rhyming echo of "ring" and "fling", as well as "string" and the more general "thing", and a contrast of direction. For whereas the stones fall downwards into the "roundy wells", the bells are "hung" (so to speak) heavenwards, like the "hung-heavenward boughs" in the poem "On the Portrait of Two Beautiful Young People".

This points to a further meaningful connection with "rounds" in "Inversnaid", as leading on "Despair to drowning". Here the "oun/own" sound suggests a movement downwards into the depths of the earth. It also recalls "The frown of his face" with "the hurtle of hell" in stanza 3 of "The Wreck". On the other hand, the downward movement is counterbalanced, if not in "Inversnaid" at least in the following poem, by an upward movement suggested by the "hung bell" as swung to and fro in the belfry so as to find "tongue to fling out broad its name".

The latter movement is significantly developed in several places in "The Wreck". One is where the poet sees the nun as "a prophetess" towering in the tumult, like the bell tower of a mediaeval church. He also listens to her "virginal tongue", as she not only "tells" but also "tolls" a divine sound of warning and comfort for the comfortless rabble. Subsequently, in stanza 31 he admires how "the breast of the maiden" could so serve as a "bell" to the "lovely-felicitous Providence" of God and "ring of it", so as to startle "the poor sheep back" to their Shepherd. This is, moreover, echoed in "The Loss of the Eurydice", with its mention of "flockbells off the aerial/ Downs' forefalls", which "beat to the burial". And the bells also serve as funeral or passing bells to convey a divine message of warning and comfort to the shipwrecked sailors.

To what now does all this point? Simply, as I have suggested, it points first downwards and then upwards. It points first, with the despair of "the leaden echo", downwards to "drowning", and then, with the hope of "the golden echo", upwards and "yonder" to the blue sky of heaven. It may be added that for Hopkins the bells themselves are not merely "hung" in belfries or church towers, but they also serve to relay to mortal ears "sunk in seeming" the soundless music of the "belled fire" of stars at night. This is precisely, as he remarks in stanza 26 of "The Wreck", "what by your measure is the heaven of desire", namely, the "azurous hung hills" which are the "world-wielding shoulder" of God himself.

Here we have the goal to which the music of Hopkins's poetry, with repeated insistence through intricate verbal echoes, is ever directing our minds. It is nothing less than the music of the spheres, the heavenly harmony from which, as Dryden says in his Song for St. Cecilia's Day (not without echoes from the music of his contemporary Henry Purcell) "this universal frame began" and which has its "closing full in man".

(*Hopkins Research* 6, July 1977)

The Two Vocations

By nature Hopkins was a poet. By divine calling and profession he was also a priest. These were his two vocations, and they are, alas, often seen as opposed to each other. But, I ask, were they really so?

To this question, as to all such difficult questions, I answer both "Yes" and "No". Yes, they were really opposed to each other, and Hopkins was right in recognizing their opposition. By nature he felt drawn to poetry, to poetic thoughts and to poetic composition. But by his sense of duty to God he was plucked away from this desire to the stern task of preparation for and exercise of the priesthood. For him, who had wished to devote his life to poetic composition, poetry could never be more than a part-time occupation or relaxation.

No doubt this constituted a strain on his life, a tension between desire and duty, between what he wanted to do and what he thought he ought to do. Yet it was for him a creative, not a destructive, tension. It was creative of all that was unique, and priestly, in his poems from "The Wreck" onwards. Had he not been a priest, Hopkins might have written more and longer and possibly (who knows?) even better poems. But he couldn't have written these poems which constitute his uniqueness as a poet for our times.

In this other sense, then, I can also answer "No". These two vocations of his weren't really opposed to each other. Rather, in their seeming opposition they come together, like fire and water in a thunderstorm, to achieve a single result. For the poems of Hopkins are more than merely religious poems, such as a layman might have written. They are priestly poems, the characteristic expressions of a priest who is a poet.

Then, what is priestly about his poems? There is, of course, a sense in which all poets are priests of a kind, particularly romantic poets. Such is the sense implied by Wordsworth, who recalls in *The Prelude* how even in his boyhood "Poetic numbers came/ Spontaneously, and clothed in priestly robe/ My spirit, thus singled out, as it might seem,/ For holy services." In this sense, the poet is a priest of nature, or rather of the divine presence in nature. By his poetic vision and composition he is a mediator between God and men, communicating to men what he has seen and offering to God what he has composed.

Hopkins, however, is a priest not only of Nature's God, but more precisely of the Christian God, Father, Son, and Holy Spirit. He looks not only, like Wordsworth, to "the dearest freshness deep down things", nor only to "the grandeur of God" with which "the world is charged", but also specifically to "the Holy Ghost" who "over the bent/ World broods with warm breast and with ah! bright wings". In this "ah!" we may recognize the climax of his poem, the moment of poetic vision and inspiration, as the poet catches in the rising of the sun a glimpse of the Holy Spirit of God.

Similarly, the poet looks up to the stars in the night sky. He points at them with intense excitement. But then he reflects on his excited feeling and finds it all too insufficient, as all too momentary. This reflection is expressed with "Ah well!" Such feelings come and go in this imperfect world of time; and yet there is something in them that doesn't come or go, something in them that depends on priestly "Prayer, patience, alms, vows". What is this something? Simply, as he says at the end of his poem, "the spouse Christ", who is shut home as it were within and behind "this piece-bright paling".

Above all, in his sonnet "Hurrahing in Harvest" Hopkins looks through the splendour and wonder of the world to the glorious mystery of the divine presence in it. Or rather, not just to the divine presence in some abstract, adjectival manner, but specifically to the presence of Christ as Saviour. So as he walks along the road on his way home, he lifts up his heart and eyes (and, no doubt, his arms, too) "Down all that glory in the heavens to glean our Saviour". He speaks to Christ, and in return he receives "a rapturous love's greeting". He is one at heart with his divine lover.

Examples might be multiplied of this Christian vision in Hopkins of the presence of God in all things, the presence of Father and Son and Holy Spirit. In this sense, he isn't just a priest of Nature, like Wordsworth, but a priest of the revelation of Grace in Nature. Yet even for this he might well have remained a Christian layman, without being an ordained priest—if a layman with an uncommon interest in theology. What in his poems then, we may ask, is so distinctive of an ordained priest?

This is to be found, I would say, not so much in his nature poems as in those which refer to human beings, inasmuch as in these poems he is prompted—as a priest— to pray for men and to offer them spiritual advice and comfort. For it belongs to a priest, as we read in the letter to the Hebrews, both to "offer up gifts and sacrifices for sins" and to "make intercession" for sinners.

The first of these functions, to pray for sinners, is abundantly illustrated in the two poems of shipwreck. One might even say that this is Hopkins's main purpose in them. In "The Wreck of the Deutschland" he admires "the call of the tall nun", as she sees Christ walking to her over the waters of affliction. At the same time, he feels "pity of the rest of them", those others who died "comfortless unconfessed", like Hamlet's poor father. He hopes that her call may have served, in God's tender providence, as a bell to "startle the poor sheep back". He also goes on to pray, through the nun's intercession, not only for her drowned fellow passengers, but for all English souls, that Christ may come back to them as King, "royally reclaiming his own".

This is also his lament and his supplication in "The Loss of the Eurydice". Deeply he deplores "These daredeaths, ay this crew, in/ Unchrist, all rolled in ruin". He is, moreover, thinking not just of their temporal but of their spiritual ruin, and not of theirs only but of the whole English race's. Bitterly he laments "The riving off that race", when the English were so cruelly cut off by their rulers from their unity with Rome and the whole of Christendom, and he grieves over the outcome of that riving which is to be seen everywhere in the land, with its "hoar-hallowed shrines unvisited". Yet all the more earnestly he prays, as a priest, "for souls sunk in seeming", and for God's "pity eternal" on them "at the awful overtaking" of the last judgment.

Nor is his prayer only for the dead, as though at some sea funeral. It is also, and much more, for the living, especially for the young, whom he regards, with a priest's eyes, with mingled hope and fear. In them he sees so much promise, though a promise that is all too often unfulfilled. This is the main purpose of his sonnet on "Spring". It isn't just to celebrate the beauty of nature at this season, but to offer up to Christ, as "maid's child", the "Innocent mind and Mayday in girl and boy", that he may preserve it "before it cloy,/ Before it cloud . . . and sour with sinning". This is, moreover, the main theme of the spiritual advice he gives from time to time, as a priest, in his poems. Just as it is the principal function of a priest to offer up sacrifices for sins, so it is the reiterated advice of this priest-poet to sacrifice all we hold most precious to God. This is what he particularly emphasizes in "Morning, Midday, and Evening Sacrifice". In the morning of life, he urges, "This, all this beauty blooming,/ This, all this freshness fuming,/ Give God while worth consuming." At midday, he continues, "This pride of prime's enjoyment/ Take as for tool, not toy meant/ And hold at Christ's employment." Finally, with renewed urgency, he ends in the evening: "What death half lifts the latch of,/ What hell hopes soon the snatch of,/ Your offering, with dispatch, of!"

To the same advice Hopkins returns, at greater length and with stronger insistence, in "The Golden Echo". There is only one way, he emphasizes, to retain "the flower of beauty, fleece of beauty", which of itself seems "too too apt to, ah! to fleet"; and that is simply to "give beauty back . . . to God", seeing that he is "beauty's self and beauty's giver". Then, as if two poems on the same subject aren't enough, he returns to it again in his sonnet "To what serves Mortal Beauty?" Here again everything leads up to the practical question, "What do then? How meet beauty?" Then with deep conviction he answers, "Merely meet it", and "Then leave, let that alone." Mortal beauty is not for mortal man, not so much because it fascinates him as because it disappoints him. It passes so swiftly, leaving him deceived and frustrated. Its true function is rather to lead men away from itself to "God's better beauty, grace".

Thus there is in Hopkins's poems something of the quality of sermons. Indeed, at more than one point we sense a hidden parallel between his poems and his sermons. Yet for a Catholic priest, in contrast to a Protestant parson, sermons are still secondary to his sacramental ministry. Even a layman may give a sermon on occasion, even from the pulpit of a Catholic church. But only the priest can administer the sacraments, chiefly those of communion, confession, and extreme unction.

The first of these three sacraments is featured in "The Bugler's First Communion". This poem isn't merely about holy communion, whether in general or on a particular occasion. It is precisely about the priest-poet's giving a boy bugler his first communion. It describes how he fetched "forth Christ from cupboard", that is, the sacred Host from the tabernacle of the altar, and how he administered "in leaf-light housel his too huge godhead", that is, Christ as truly present in the seeming wafer of bread. "There!"—so swiftly and easily. The rest of the poem is a prayer for the lad, and for the well working of "that sealing sacred ointment" which he has received at baptism and confirmation.

Complementary to this poem of first communion is the poet's moving description of his administration of the last sacraments to "Felix Randal the farrier". He recalls how their heavenly effect was realized in him "some/ Months earlier, since I had our sweet reprieve and ransom/ Tendered to him". Not only did he then bring him communion after confession, with (possibly) the sacrament of extreme unction, but he also comforted him with his tongue and quenched his tears with his touch. And those tears that then so touched his heart continue to touch the hearts of his readers.

There is yet another way in which Hopkins was a priest in his poetry. It is a way even more essential to his priesthood than the administration of the sacraments. I mean the way of sacrifice, not just in moral exhortation or sacramental administration, but in personal experience. This is the way we find, above all, in the dark sonnets of his later, Dublin years.

The darkness of these sonnets is basically a sacrificial darkness, deeply affecting one who is, like Christ on the cross, both priest and victim. Before, the poet was more conscious of his sacramental and spiritual priesthood. Now, he is made aware by bitter experience of the sacrificial nature of a priest as victim. As he laments in one of the sonnets, he is cut off as by a sword of parting from "father and mother dear", from "brothers and sisters", and from England as "wife to my creating thought", not just in a physical but in a spiritual sense for the sake of Christ. Yet this is only the beginning of his sacrifice. Part of it, too, was no doubt his personal decision to renounce poetic composition on entering religious life in the Society of Jesus. Even though he qualified this renunciation by the saving clause "unless it were by the wish of my superior", he was obliged by his circumstances as a priest to renounce the fame of a poet during his lifetime. This is a cause of his feeling of bitter frustration, which he goes on to utter in his above-mentioned sonnet: "Only what word/ Wisest my heart breeds, dark heaven's baffling ban/ Bars or hell's spell thwarts. This to hoard unheard,/ Heard unheeded, leaves me a lonely began."

Paradoxically this priestly sacrifice of Hopkins consists in his being cut off not only from his fellow men, but even from God himself. As priest and mediator between God and men, he has not only to be in communication with the one and the other. He must also suffer a strange separation from the one and the other. Thus it was that Christ himself on the cross cried out to his Father, "My God, my God, why have you abandoned me?" Similarly Hopkins complains, "And my lament/ Is cries countless, cries like dead letters sent/ To dearest him that lives alas! away." All he can do in his suffering is to exhort himself to bear it all with patience, though patience is "the hard thing", even to pray or bid for. Yet it is through patience, rather than prayer, that as a priest the poet comes closest to God. For God, too, "is patient". And it is by his experience of suffering that, as a priest-poet, Hopkins can preach patience to his suffering fellow men.

In all these ways Hopkins contrived to practise his priesthood not in spite of, but by means of, his poetry. He couldn't remain content with two departments in his life, the one as it were sealed off from the other, the one for professional duty, the other for pleasure and relaxation. For that would have been a narrowing of his ideal of the priesthood, on the one hand, and a degrading of his view of poetry, on the other. After all, the priesthood isn't just a profession to be exercised at stated times. It involves the whole man and enters into all his activities, whether of an explicitly priestly nature or not. Nor is poetry a mere pastime for pleasure or relaxation from higher duties. It has a high nobility of its own.

Hopkins then succeeded in fusing the two together in a personal synthesis of his own; and the outcome of the resulting tension was the unique creation of a new kind of poetry endowed with his priestly character. In it he not only preached sacrifice to others. He also offered the sacrifice of himself in a spirit of prayer and patience through Christ as "hero of Calvary" to the eternal Father.

(*Hopkins Research* 7, August 1978)

The Poems of 1879

WHAT ARE "the poems of 1879"? Is there anything special characterizing them and differentiating them from Hopkins's other poems? From a merely extrinsic viewpoint, they are the few poems he composed during his year's ministry on the staff of St. Aloysius's church at Oxford from December 1878 till October 1879. They thus represent his impressions on returning to Oxford as a Jesuit priest after an absence of over twenty years from his graduation in 1867. But there is something more to them than just this extrinsic viewpoint.

The first two of these poems, "Binsey Poplars" and "Duns Scotus's Oxford", are explicitly about Oxford and its rural setting, "rounded" by the river. The poet is evidently glad to be back in the university of his favourite philosopher, "Of realty the rarest-veined unraveller", who has taught him to recognize the *haecceitas* or *ecceitas*, the unique individuality of things—or that in them which makes us refer to them as "this" and which makes us exclaim, "*Ecce!* Behold!" At the same time he is saddened at the newly arisen "base and brickish skirt" which now confounds the "rural keeping" of the city. Even more deeply he is saddened at the "strokes of havoc" on the familiar line of poplar trees that used to grow by the river bank near Binsey, so as to "unselve the sweet especial scene".

Thus from the outset these two poems indicate the main emphasis of the poet's mind in this year at Oxford, an emphasis which continues into his next poem, "Henry Purcell". Here one finds no special connection with Oxford, apart from the word "special", or rather "arch-especial". What Hopkins has so admired in the philosophy of Scotus he finds practically illustrated in the music of Purcell, with his "arch-especial spirit" and "the rehearsal of own, of abrupt self" which "so thrusts on, so throngs the ear".

Comparing these three poems with one another, one may further notice a movement from the celebration of natural beauty and its lamentable ruin in "Binsey Poplars" and "Duns Scotus's Oxford" to that of man and the human spirit in "Henry Purcell". This may correspond to the fact that at Oxford the poet found himself more in contact with man than with nature, in the form not now of university students but of the parishioners and altar boys at St. Aloysius'.

It is for this reason that in the next three poems of this year there is a distinctly personal emphasis both in their subjective style and in their objective content. First, there is the vaguer "Candle Indoors", echoing the previous "Lantern out of Doors". Here the poet presents himself as passing outside a lighted window one night and wondering "what task what fingers ply" there. His attention is, however, occupied not so much by the personal selves of "Jessy or Jack", who remain unindividualized, as by his own self, his "first and vital candle in close heart's vault".

In the next poem, however, he is drawn out of himself in admiration of "The Handsome Heart" revealed in the "gracious answer" of one of his altar boys. Dwelling on the delicate manners of the boy, in response to the offer of a reward, the poet notes, first, the "wild and self-instressed" quality of "homing nature", and then, completing the work of nature, the higher work of "hallowing grace". At the same time he can't merely dwell on the present, but as a priest he must needs look forward to the future and exhort the boy to effort and sacrifice: "O brace sterner that strain!"

The same movement, not only from nature to man, but also from natural beauty in man to divine grace, with an accompanying need of effort and sacrifice, appears in "The Bugler's First Communion". Here the poet moves as it were from the sacristy, where he presumably spoke with the altar boy, to the church, where he gives his first communion to a boy bugler. He is impressed by the "bloom of a chastity in mansex fine", which "hies headstrong to its well-being of a self-wise self-will". At the same time he expresses his concern for the future, his fear of disappointment in "those sweet hopes" and his prayer to "favourable heaven".

His emphasis on sacrifice and renunciation of "mortal beauty" comes to a climax in the next poem, entitled "Morning, Midday, and Evening Sacrifice". Not only in childhood, he insists, but throughout life beauty must be offered to God "while worth consuming", since only God can keep it from being consumed. In this process of sacrifice he distinguishes three main phases. First comes the morning of "all this beauty blooming" in youth. Then there is the midday, or "pride of prime's enjoyment" in manhood, followed by the evening of "mastery in the mind". Here is a fundamental theme, namely the necessary conjunction of beauty and sacrifice, which the poet goes on to develop in two later poems, "The Leaden Echo and the Golden Echo" and "To what serves Mortal Beauty?"

Finally, we come to two sonnets that express the poet's deepening anxiety both for the Church in the contemporary world and for himself. The Church he sees in "Andromeda" in terms of the classical legend of Perseus and Andromeda. Perseus for him is Christ, and Andromeda is the Church "on this rock rude", unequalled as well in beauty as in injury. As for himself, he feels in his other "curtal" sonnet on "Peace" how much he stands in need of the Spirit of Peace, whom he compares to a "wild wooddove". Common to both these sonnets is the theme of patience. With regard to the Church, he speaks of "her patience, morselled into pangs". In himself, too, he looks to "Patience exquisite,/ That plumes to Peace thereafter". In all this, moreover, he looks implicitly to the dark sonnets of his later years, culminating in that on "Patience".

In this way, we may find in all these poems of 1879 a kind of turning point from the bright sonnets of the St. Beuno's period (1874–77) to the dark sonnets of the Dublin period (1884–89). In them we find a movement from nature to man, from the men around the poet to his own self, from the desire for mortal beauty to the perceived need of sacrifice and renunciation. At the same time, both within and above them all is the poet's religious motive of praise and service directed to God through Christ our Lord in the Spirit of Peace and Love.

(*Hopkins Research* 8, September 1979)

"*Spring and Fall*", 1980

We live today in an age of the celebration of anniversaries, not least literary anniversaries. Considering how rich is the history of English literature, it isn't surprising that each year brings a fresh batch of centenaries calling for celebration. Usually, and rightly, we think in terms of the births and deaths of mortal men. But occasionally, we do well to remember the births of their immortal works. Not so long ago, in the case of Hopkins, we were recalling the birth of his immortal poem, "The Wreck of the Deutschland"; and now I see no reason why we shouldn't go on to recall the births of his subsequent, if shorter, poems one by one, year after year. So in this year of 1980 we may well turn to that most charming of his poems, "Spring and Fall", and pause a while in contemplation of its deceptive simplicity.

Among all the poems of Hopkins this is outstanding for its paradoxical combination of simplicity and profundity. Its simplicity is seen, or better heard, in what the poet says. Its profundity is not so much seen or heard as understood or dimly perceived in what he doesn't say, or refuses to say.

To begin with, this poem is so refreshingly simple, in contrast to the endless complications and convolutions of

Hopkins's other poems from "The Wreck of the Deutschland" onwards. Even his friend Bridges, so obtuse with regard to his other poems, could hardly remain obtuse to this. It consists almost entirely of Teutonic monosyllables; and even the two disyllables, "wanwood" and "leafmeal", which call for some elucidation, are Teutonic and fall without difficulty into their component parts. The sentences are short, and the syntax is unusually straightforward. The metre, too, is of the simplest: tetrameter, with a strongly pronounced beat, partly conversational, partly incantational, that here and there contains just a suggestion of sprung rhythm.

Why, I would like to ask, is this poem so simple, in contrast to the other poems of Hopkins? Why has he here departed from his customary complexity? In answer to this question I would like to offer three reasons, not distinct from each other, but leading from one to the other and together coalescing to form a coherent unity.

First comes the fact that in this year Hopkins, as a Jesuit priest, was attached to the parish staff of St. Francis Xavier's church in Liverpool. There the people he had to deal with, and preach to, were rougher and simpler than those he met at his previous positions in London and Oxford. He could hardly speak to them with the metaphysical subtlety of a Duns Scotus, but he must needs descend to their plebeian, plain-spoken, matter-of-fact level. Not that their plainness was alien to his refined, aesthetic taste. For all the sophistication of his literary and philosophical culture, there had always been in him a hankering for the simplicity of childhood and the wanton wildness of boyhood. Even his theological training had been carried out to the accompaniment of the Gregorian chant or plainsong, which (as he later admitted to Canon Dixon) was now in his mind during the composition of this poem.

Secondly, and more particularly, there is the added fact that in this poem Hopkins is speaking—or rather, imagining himself speaking—"to a young child". It may not, as he told Bridges, have been founded on any real incident, but it was surely based on a generic concept of the children he found in the parish of St. Francis Xavier's, and crystallized in the form of a little girl to whom he gives the enchanting name of Margaret. Perhaps he recalled the memory of a child—it may even have been himself—weeping bitterly over the falling leaves of autumn, as he walked along the country road near Lydiate just outside Liverpool that day in early September 1880. Perhaps, too, he was thinking of all the criticisms of oddity levelled against him by his friend Bridges; and perhaps it occurred to him that the best way of avoiding them would be to address a poem to a child, preferably a little girl, who would be more sensitive to such natural phenomena than a little boy.

Thirdly, and paradoxically, there is the profound thought of the poem, which I think best explains its simplicity. With all his metaphysical subtlety, following in the footsteps of the Subtle Doctor, Hopkins recognized and adored the divine Word in the form of an infant, the *Verbum abbreviatum*, or Word foredrawn and adapted to the slender capacity of the human understanding. Human words, however multiplied and elaborated and distinguished, fail to express divine truth or divine mystery in its fullness. On the other hand, it is not infrequently the failure of human words in a moment of tension that reveals something of this truth or mystery in the ensuing silence—in the form of what is technically known as aposiopesis.

This is what Hopkins has already hinted in "The Wreck", speaking of himself in words that he subsequently echoes in this poem: "Ah, touched in your bower of bone,/ Are you!

Turned for an exquisite smart,/ Have you! Make words break from me here all alone,/ Do you!" Then, when he comes to give more precise expression to this "exquisite smart", he finds the words themselves breaking in the climactic moment of vision: "But how shall I . . . make me room there:/ Reach me a . . . Fancy, come faster—/ Strike you the sight of it? Look at it loom there,/ Thing that she . . . there then! the Master." Here words are plainly inadequate to utter what the poet, or the nun, sees. Yet their very inadequacy strangely serves to utter it.

So it is here, too, in "Spring and Fall". At every point in the poem something is falling, something is breaking, something is silent. The leaves are falling from the trees of Goldengrove, leaving "worlds of wanwood leafmeal" on the ground. The heart of the young child is grieving, even breaking into sobs and tears, over the falling leaves. The one is a reflection of the other—"leaves, like the things of man". Together they point to a mystery that is hidden in "sorrow's springs". For adults, in whom reason is more fully developed, in "the light of common day", the mystery remains hidden. But children, with their "fresh thoughts", can at least perceive it, even if they can't understand or name it.

So the poet appropriately comes to the heart of the mystery with a series of negatives that serve not so much to comfort the child as to deepen her grief with the added sense of mystery. Even while refusing to name it, "Now no matter, child, the name", he touches on the thing itself. Even while declaring the inadequacy of mouth and mind, "Nor mouth had, no nor mind expressed", he points to a possibility of perception in the heart and inmost spirit of man. What is this perception? Prudently the poet doesn't say, though he seems to know it. All he will say, considering the capacity of the child, is that "It is the blight man was born for", the curse of what she will come to know as "original sin" as she grows older. Or rather, to put it more simply and more profoundly, "It is Margaret you mourn for."

Who then, we may finally ask, is speaking? Who is telling all these riddles to this little girl? It is, of course, the poet, speaking in the form of tetrameter with rhyming couplets. But in this poem he is, more than in his other poems, more than a mere poet: He is also a priest and a preacher. And this young child, Margaret, is his parishioner and congregation. He is preaching to her, and giving her spiritual advice, not out of his superior wisdom as an adult, but out of that Word of God which has been entrusted to him by his priestly ordination. It is his vocation and his duty not only to preach that Word, but also to adapt it to the mind and capacity of his congregation. And when the congregation is (representatively) "a young child", he must provide what St. Paul calls not meat for grown men but milk for babes.

So in this poem we may see the poet's consummate abbreviation of his various meditations on the divine Word, as received from the pages of Holy Scripture according to the traditional teaching of the Catholic Church. From the depths of his heart he speaks to the heart of this young child and utters not only his own sounding words as man but also something of the silent Word of God.

(*Hopkins Research* 9, July 1980)

The Worst of Hopkins

THE LAST THREE lines of the dark sonnet "I wake and feel", which Hopkins revised not once but many times, lead up none the less to a monumental crux: "Selfyeast of spirit a dull dough sours. I see/ The lost are like this, and their scourge to be/ As I am mine, their sweating selves; but worse."

To begin with, there seems to be an ambiguity concerning the subject and object of "sours" in the first line. Only, in this case we are aided by an earlier version of the line, "by selfyeast so soured", where it is evidently "selfyeast" that does the souring and the "dull dough" of the body that is soured. Here the poet was presumably revising not his meaning, so as to make it more ambiguous, but his wording, so as to make it more varied in sound and more tense in structure.

The real crux, however, comes in the last line, and in the last word of that line, where an ambiguity still remains, for all the poet's revising, in the unexpressed subject of "worse". Here there seem to be two possibilities. It is either the "I" of "I see" or the "the lost" of "The lost are like this". Even if we look for guidance to the previous version, "Their sweating selves as I am mine, but worse", we come up against the same ambiguity. All the poet has done to his first version is to shift the position of "as I am mine" to the beginning of the line and to alter the comma before "but" to a semi-colon. In either case there remains not only an ambiguity, to enrich the meaning in an Empsonian sense, but also the dark possibility of a heretical interpretation. That is to say, in comparing himself to the damned in hell, Hopkins dares to suggest that his pains are "worse" than theirs. Even if this is only one of two opposite interpretations, the fact remains that the poet, for all his revising, has allowed it to stand.

Traditionally, Hopkins scholars follow the orthodox interpretation in their commentaries on this line. After all, they reflect, Hopkins was a dutiful and devout Jesuit priest, whose theological orthodoxy stands out in all his sermons and other spiritual writings. He would hardly have strayed from orthodoxy in this one passage, even in such a dark sonnet as "I wake and feel", as to imply that his momentary pains on earth could be worse than the eternal pains of the damned in hell. It would have been contrary to his known character, particularly as expressed in his reaction to the temptation of Despair in "Carrion Comfort", to say so. Hence, even if he has left the wording of this last line of "I wake and feel" open to a heterodox interpretation, we may well resolve the ambiguity in the light of his prevailing orthodox belief and conclude that it must be "the lost" who are "worse".

On the other hand, the opposite conclusion is strongly maintained by one commentator on this poem, Daniel A. Harris, in his *Inspirations Unbidden* (Berkeley, 1982). Dismissing the traditional interpretation as "a common misreading", he maintains that "neither the grammatical structure of the tercet nor the evidence of Hopkins's revisions" supports it. In other, plainer words, the speaker, so far from believing himself redeemed by Christ and recognizing the lot of the damned as worse than his own, "considers himself beyond redemption, cannot make the 'turn' to Christ, and thus comes perilously close to sinning against the divine omnipotence".

If this is indeed what the poet considers, then he is leaving himself open to the serious charge of heresy. But, I ask, is this really what the poet considers? Or is it only what the author thinks the poet considers? How does the author prove what he thinks? It isn't enough for him to speak of the poet's meaning behind his words, as if he is gifted with an insight beyond other readers. It is necessary for him to show how this meaning, and (as Harris maintains) only this meaning, is embedded in the words of the poem. So to support his assertion, Harris proposes two arguments based on the words of the poem; and these call for our careful attention, one by one.

In the first place, he asserts, Hopkins's introduction of the semicolon before "but worse" produces in that fragmentary sentence a grammatical structure parallel to "I see . . .", that is, "but (I am) worse". But, I ask, does it produce such a grammatical structure? If one assumes the ellipsis of "I am" after "but", there certainly appears to be a parallelism between "I see" and "but (I am) worse". But do we really have to assume this ellipsis? Isn't there another possible ellipsis, "but (they are) worse"? This also leaves a good grammatical structure within the clause that follows on "I see". In this case, it is true, the clause is divided in two by a semicolon, which may make things grammatically difficult. But from the viewpoint of prosody (which was for Hopkins of far more importance than grammar) we may consider that "I see" comes at the end of the twelfth line and thus serves to introduce all that follows in the next two lines. In this case, it is more prosodically natural for "but worse" to follow on "The lost are like this" than on "I see".

Now, to return from considerations of grammar and prosody to those of theological meaning, the last two words, "but worse", may be interpreted as an afterthought of the poet for the sake of orthodoxy. After all, he has just been comparing his condition to that of the damned in hell. But he can't simply leave it at that, for it might savour of heresy. There is a difference, he can't help admitting, between his mental condition, however desperate it may feel, and that of the damned. At least, as his Catholic faith assures him, however deeply he feels his sweating self, he remains in this world of time, where all is comparative and nothing as yet superlative. For him there is as yet "no worst". That is the lot of those who are lost forever, who have to suffer the torment of hell forever. However much he may suffer, he isn't yet one of those lost, though he may feel his torment resembling theirs. In this respect at least, namely, "the pain of loss", which is forever, their torment must be judged "worse" than his.

Secondly, Harris discerns a syntactical interweaving between the speaker and the damned in what he calls "a pattern of alternation that generates a primary awareness of sameness, not of difference". This pattern he displays by italicising Hopkins's words in the following manner: "*their* scourge to be/ as I am mine,/ *their* sweating selves;/ but (I am) worse." But, I ask again, is this pattern of alternation implicit in Hopkins's words? Or is it merely what Kant would call a "subjective form" in Harris's mind? For there is another alternative we have to consider. In the traditional interpretation, "but (they are) worse", there is a pattern not of alternation, which is somewhat tame and unlike Hopkins, but of contrast, not unlike the pattern in sprung rhythm. Normally perhaps one might expect the pattern ABAB, which is what "alternation" means. But when the less expected pattern ABAA occurs, by "contrast", it serves to bring out the final A all the more strongly, and so to reaffirm the poet's orthodoxy.

In these two answers to the two "proofs" advocated by Harris, however, I do not claim to have refuted his interpretation. I claim no more than to have refuted his assertion that his is the only correct interpretation and that the other is a "common misreading". I claim no more than to have shown that this other has at least as much right to be accepted as a valid interpretation, in view both of the final and of the previous version of the lines in question. So to decide which of the two interpretations is the better, or even the only acceptable one, we have to take into account not only the grammar and prosody of the lines but also the prevailing mind of the poet, as we find it not only in his spiritual writings of the period but also in the poems composed before and after this one. And about his prevailing mind, there can surely be no doubt about the poet's orthodoxy till the end.

Still, there remains one more argument of a syntactical nature which I ought to mention, as it seems to have escaped Harris's notice altogether. I mean the evident parallelism of the two sonnets "No worst" and "I wake and feel". From the beginning of the latter poem we find an apparent continuity with the former, even though they are separated in the customary sequence (based on Hopkins's own MS) by "To seem the stranger". For whereas the poet ended the former with the cold comfort, supplied by Shakespeare, that "All life death does end and each day dies with sleep", he now feels himself deprived even of that comfort, and so he declares, "I wake and feel the fell of dark, not day." On the other hand, whereas he began the former with the despairing cry, also supplied by Shakespeare, "No worst, there is none", he now comes upon a further comfort, even in comparing his condition with that of the lost, inasmuch as "their scourge" is "worse". Thus in the end of the latter poem he reaffirms what he said at the beginning of the former, but with a new emphasis. For out of the despair of "No worst (for me)" he paradoxically draws the hope of "but worse (than mine)".

This comfort we may surely be allowed, in spite of Harris's determination to rub our noses (and that of Hopkins) in the dust of misery, to see steadily growing in the sonnets that follow. We may see it, for example, in the "root-room" afforded by his exhortation to "patience", in his profession of faith in the "delicious kindness" of God, recalling the "lovely-felicitous Providence" of "The Wreck" (st.31), and in his vision of the divine "smile" which so suddenly and unexpectedly "lights a lovely mile". If we accept this sequence as both natural (to the mind of Hopkins) and chronological (to his pen), we may well go on to recognize how aptly "That Nature is a Heraclitean Fire" comes three years later as a climax to Hopkins's testing during those years "of now done darkness".

In this poem, Harris protests, "the need for apocalypse is so pressing that the speaker, without preparation, simply asserts its sudden happening". On the contrary, I say, everything Hopkins ever wrote, everything he believed, leads up to this moment. Everything in his life and work, for anyone who has eyes to see, appears in the light of this poem as having been a preparation not, as Socrates saw his life, for death but, as Hopkins learnt from the teaching of Christ, for resurrection and eternal life.

(*Hopkins Research* 12, November 1983)

Hopkins's "Comfort"

THERE ARE MANY WAYS of interpreting the long sonnet of 1888 to which Hopkins gave the appropriately long title, "That Nature is a Heraclitean Fire and of the comfort of the Resurrection". One way is to concentrate on the one noun in this title which is left, somewhat unexpectedly, uncapitalized and to ask the question "Why?" Why is this most important word left without the capital C, while Nature, the Heraclitean Fire, and the Resurrection all receive their due of capitalization? An obvious answer is that these other nouns are all treated as proper names: the goddess Nature, the Fire as the outward form of the divine Logos according to the theory of Heraclitus, and the Resurrection of Christ, who told Martha, "I am the Resurrection and the Life." On the other hand, "comfort" is the only common noun among them, though not for that reason of no significance. It may be lacking in the "this-ness" of those proper names, but it may well merit our attention as their servant, whose function it is to bring out their significance.

To begin with, the phrase, "the comfort of the Resurrection", serves to indicate that the poem embodies the poet's answer to his previous frantic questioning, "Comforter, where, where is your comforting?" This is the question to which he had been looking in vain for an answer in the course of his dark sonnets, casting for comfort "by groping round my comfortless" room. The only outcome of his search had been his weary advice to his "poor Jackself" to cease tormenting himself, to "call off thoughts awhile/ Elsewhere" and to "leave comfort root-room". But that is easier said than done, even within the rigid restrictions of the sonnet form. For beyond these restrictions his questioning cannot but continue, with the further question, "If elsewhere, then where?" Where, but in that world of Nature, which had been the subject of his bright sonnets, though in the dark sonnets it had been replaced by a tormenting preoccupation with his "soul, self . . . poor Jackself"?

The turning point for that change, from bright to dark, appears in what Hopkins calls "the longest sonnet ever made", namely, "Spelt from Sibyl's Leaves". There he presents the world of Nature as changing from the light of day to the darkness of night, in terms not of an objective landscape, such as we find in Gray's "Elegy", but of a subjective inscape all his own, if we may use that poetic term in a less technical sense. There he exclaims, "Our evening is over us; our night whelms, whelms, and will end us." It is the evening that introduces the dark night of the dark sonnets, in which the being not only of Nature but even of Self seems at an end.

But no! By leaving "comfort root-room", by letting "joy size at God knows when to God knows what", by allowing "natural heart's ivy, Patience" to mask his "ruins of wrecked past purpose", the poet comes to realize the lesson that Nature, and Nature's God, is always trying to teach him, namely, the lesson of transformation. Evening may move into night, as "the last lights off the black West went"; but in a little while, with patience and the passing of time, "Oh, morning, at the brown brink eastward, springs." The one follows the other, as Polonius pompously tells his son Laertes, "as the night the day". The light of day may be swallowed up by the darkness of night; but the night is in turn dissipated by the rising of a new day. Thus in Nature "everything goes by contraries". And thus, in the poetic composition of Hopkins, just as the dark sonnets are ushered in by what he then calls "the longest sonnet ever made", so they are ushered out by an even longer sonnet with a title incorporating the keyword "comfort".

The view of Nature which provides the poet with his point of departure in this poem is one suggested by his long familiarity with early Greek philosophy, particularly the cryptic fragments of Heraclitus. This he announces in the first half of his title, with reference to the "Heraclitean Fire". But the poem is more than a distillation of "a great deal of early Greek philosophical thought", as the poet explains to his friend Bridges. It is also evidently inspired by his "remembrance of things past", including his own previous poems. Thus he seems to recall "Inversnaid" in "cloud-puffball, torn tufts", "Hurrahing in Harvest" in "an air-built thoroughfare", "Carrion Comfort" in "ropes, wrestles, beats earth bare", "God's Grandeur" in "squandering ooze" and "treadmire toil", and above all "The Wreck of the Deutschland" in such words as "lace", "wrestles", "yestertempest", "dust", "stanches", and "million-fueled". More immediately, however, the poet is inspired, as in "Hurrahing in Harvest", by the weather of a particular day in Dublin, "one windy bright day between floods", as he describes it in a letter to Canon Dixon, in "a preposterous summer". The inspiration of that day, combined with his remembrance of past poems and "early Greek philosophical thought", serves to tide him over the octet and into the ninth line of the sonnet.

But then, like Hamlet, he finds his inspiration suddenly checked by "the pale cast of thought", expressed here in the form of a "but", introducing Death as the opponent of Nature in all living creatures but especially in Man. "But quench," he says, with an echo both of Othello's soliloquy previous to his murder of Desdemona and of the other soliloquy he himself put into the mouth of Caradoc after the murder of St. Winefred. That is what Death does to the "clearest-selved spark" in Nature, namely Man, thereby destroying what is loveliest in mortal beauty. Such is the consideration that plunges the poet back into the despairing thoughts of his dark sonnets, with a return to that "vaulty, voluminous . . . stupendous evening" in "Spelt from Sibyl's Leaves", as he ponders the "unfathomable . . . enormous dark" when "vastness blurs and time beats level" the memory of Man. This consideration, moreover, carries the poet well beyond the limits of the sestet, and of the sonnet form, with one and a half more lines of a coda—till as suddenly as he has entered into it, he brings himself to a halt with an unexpected "Enough!"

Yes, this "Enough!" is unexpected in terms of this particular poem, but it isn't so unexpected in terms of the poet's output or his life as a whole. We even find the same turn of phrase in his previous unfinished poem, "On the Portrait of Two Beautiful Young People" (dated 1886), whose final stanza begins, "Enough: corruption was the world's first woe." Only, in the present poem Hopkins turns from "Enough" not to "corruption" but to "the Resurrection" (with a capital R), by way of synthesis to the foregoing antithesis. He also looks back from the "grief's gasping, joyless days, dejection" of the dark sonnets to the abiding memory of the bright sonnets and, above all, of "The Wreck of the Deutschland". Now, more than ever before, he identifies himself with the drowning nun in his experience of being "in an enormous dark drowned"; and out of this darkness he sees Christ coming to him as his "heart's light" and "a blown beacon of light". Indeed, at this point in the poem everything seems to come back to him out of that supremely creative moment in his past, as he looks (so to say) from the wreck to "The Wreck". On the one hand, he is troubled by his "foundering deck", the falling of flesh and "world's wildfire", with everything approaching its fated end. But on the other hand, he is comforted by "a beacon, an eternal beam", which appears to him "in a flash, at a trumpet crash . . . all at once", recalling "as once at a crash Paul" from "The Wreck".

This is, to be sure, not what one would expect in the order of Nature, even in the sense implied by Shelley, where he speaks in his "Ode to the West Wind" of the "clarion" of Spring. Rather, with his "Enough!", Hopkins suddenly flees "with a fling of the heart", as he had fled in "The Wreck", from the order of Nature to that of Grace and towers "from the grace to the Grace". This is the deep impulse of his Christian faith, which is entirely characteristic of him and his poems, at least from "The Wreck" onwards. It is precisely this leap of faith, which both looks to and reflects the Resurrection, that imparts to the poems of Hopkins their characteristic dynamism—"the roll, the rise, the carol, the creation", which he fears missing from his final poem, "To R. B.", the following year. Here it is fully present, for those who have ears to hear it, in the "heart's clarion" and the "trumpet crash"—where one may also discern an echo from Browning's "Rabbi Ben Ezra": "The festal board, lamp's flash and trumpet's peal."

Thus it is that the poet is enabled to make his way, more fully than ever before, "to hero of Calvary, Christ's feet", as he recollects how "he was what I am". In this recollection, moreover, he discovers the supreme rhyme of his eccentric prosody between "I am, and" and "diamond". By this discovery he is also enabled to effect a poetic transformation, analogous to that awaiting realization in the final resurrection, from "this Jack, joke, poor potsherd, patch, matchwood, immortal diamond" to what is purely "immortal diamond". That is to say, what precedes the change is merely a miscellaneous conglomeration of conflicting qualities, most of them worthless and destined to be purged away, but one of them endowed with infinite value as (in the words of Shakespeare) an "eternal jewel"; whereas what follows is the manifestation of what is best in himself and, in fact, "what in God's eye he is—Christ".

Now at last, we may say in conclusion, the poet encounters that divine smile which, as he rightly foresees—even in the midst of his dark night, "as skies/ Betweenpie mountains—lights a lovely mile" for the last year of his life on earth. Now at last he finds "the comfort of the Resurrection", which is not to be "wrung" by an artificial violence from above but to be drawn up from the depths of his Christian faith. Only, in his faith and humility he prefers to spell that "comfort" with a small letter, recognizing with St. Paul that what he feels on earth "as it were in a glass darkly" isn't to be compared with that true Comfort (spelt with a capital letter) which remains to be revealed in heaven.

(*Hopkins Research* 13, July 1984)

Hopkinsian Reminiscences

Hopkins was born and brought up in London: so was I. Hopkins went up to Oxford, to study the Classics: so did I. Hopkins decided to enter the Society of Jesus: so did I. Hopkins spent the years of his Jesuit formation at Manresa, Stonyhurst, and St. Beuno's: so did I. Hopkins lived three years at St. Beuno's and went on a pilgrimage to St. Winefred's Well: so did I. Hopkins spent summer vacations at Barmouth on the Welsh coast, and went on a rowing trip to Penmaenpool: so did I. After his ordination to the priesthood, Hopkins stayed at such places as Mount St. Mary's, Farm Street, and St. Aloysius' Oxford: so have I. Hopkins was sent to teach literature at a university overseas: so was I. During his exile Hopkins wrote "terrible sonnets": so have I.

Such is the preface I sometimes make at the beginning of a course of lectures on the poetry of Hopkins, by way of self-introduction. It gives my students some assurance that I can speak on this subject as an "insider"; but more importantly, it all leads up to the humorous anti-climax, which Hopkins himself might have enjoyed with his delight in puns. For I, too, have composed not a few sonnets in my Japanese exile; and I expect that not a few critics, if they came across them, would dismiss them as "terrible"—though in a different sense from that applied to the dark sonnets of Hopkins. After all, I might add, my experience of teaching literature in exile has been very different from, in the sense of having been far more enjoyable than, that of Hopkins.

Now let me go back and attempt an answer to the question, when and how I first discovered the poetry of Hopkins. Oddly enough, for all the parallels I have just drawn between Hopkins and myself, I didn't really discover his poetry till I came to Japan. Till then I had merely been aware of his name and the fact that he had composed some odd, unintelligible poems, which only odd, unintelligible people, the sort of people who are regarded by the English as "intellectuals", went in for.

Even in my boyhood at the Jesuit college of Wimbledon, I had been aware of his existence in connection with an old, eccentric priest there, named Geoffrey Bliss. Father Bliss was himself something of a poet; and he had been one of the earliest promoters of Hopkins's poetry after the Great War (as we then called the First World War). His name appears in not a few Hopkins bibliographies. But he had no influence on my boyhood, at least in any poetical sense. I regarded him only as an old priest to be avoided when it came to serving morning Mass at the Sacred Heart church, he was so eccentric and rough with small boys.

Even when I left school to join the Jesuit noviceship at St. Beuno's College in 1943, it hardly entered my mind that this was the place where Hopkins had studied theology and composed "The Wreck of the Deutschland". Nor did our master of novices ever allude to the fact. We were just not interested. Two years later, when I took my first vows and stayed on at St. Beuno's for my first year of juniorate, it was only to have been expected that in our study of literature we should have been introduced to the poetry of Hopkins. But no! Even then Hopkins made no impact on my mind. During that year we spent a pleasant summer vacation at Hodder Place, near Stonyhurst, and I was deeply impressed by the mountain scenery. But I never knew how carefully it had all been described by Hopkins in his Notebooks.

Then for my second year of juniorate, I went to Manresa House, Roehampton, to the southwest of London, where Hopkins had spent his noviceship and later taught the classics to the juniors. But still I was unaware of his presence or his influence. For the next three years, from 1947 to 1950, I studied scholastic philosophy at Heythrop College in the wilds of Oxfordshire, far from Hopkinsian haunts, since Hopkins had made his study of philosophy at St. Mary's Hall, Stonyhurst, where I had been only for the summer in my first year of juniorate. While I was there, even Oxford seemed far away, and it was chiefly associated in our minds with visits to the doctor or the dentist. During this time, however, I also, like Hopkins, conceived an interest in the philosophy of Duns Scotus, though I could hardly say that I was, like Hopkins, "flush with a new stroke of enthusiasm". In any case, my interest was purely philosophical and not at all literary, and quite unconnected with any influence from Hopkins.

It was then that, like Hopkins, I went with the other "philosophers" (as we students of scholastic philosophy were called) for our summer vacation to Barmouth. And from Barmouth, on a special day called "the George Day", we all went on a rowing expedition up the estuary of the river Mawddach to the George Inn at Penmaenpool for lunch, and then rowed back with the outgoing tide in the afternoon. On one such occasion we were joined by a young American Jesuit priest, Father Anthony Bischoff, who was (it seemed to us) quite nuts on Gerard Manley Hopkins. He had come all the way to join us, just to see the very place where Hopkins had composed his rather inferior poem entitled "Penmaen Pool". "How ridiculous!" we thought—though politeness and prudence prevented us from giving expression to our thoughts in his hearing.

Another American Jesuit, Father Raymond Schoder, whom I met about this time, had come to England for much the same purpose—though it was professedly for his year of tertianship at St. Beuno's. We also regarded him as mildly crazy for the photos he insisted on taking of places in the British Isles connected with the person and the poems of Hopkins. While he was at St. Beuno's, I was informed, he would hang out of trees at the most impossible angles in order to get the best view of the college for his camera. He even journeyed to Harwich on the Essex coast to take another picture of the exact spot where the *Deutschland* had foundered in 1875, though, as it was only the sea, it might have been anywhere!

From Heythrop I went up to Oxford in 1950, not, of course, to Balliol College (where Hopkins had spent his undergraduate years), nor to the Jesuit church of St. Aloysius (where Hopkins had served on the staff), but to the Jesuit house of studies, Campion Hall. There for the next four years I devoted myself to the study first (like Hopkins) of the classics, then (unlike Hopkins) of English literature. Now I might have been expected to include Hopkins's poems in my study of English, especially as his poems and prose writings had all been published by the Oxford University Press. But again, no! The obligatory papers in English extended only up to the romantic poets, and I didn't care to choose the optional paper (for an additional examination) on Victorian literature. And even if I had included

Victorian literature in my choice of papers, Hopkins wasn't yet the "must" he became in subsequent years.

During my time at Oxford, when I walked to Binsey in the summer term, I was drawn not so much by the line of poplars—which are still there, in spite of having been felled while Hopkins was at St. Aloysius's—as by the sight of sailing boats on the river. Again, when I went to St. Aloysius's church, it was mostly to act as subdeacon for High Mass on Sunday, without ever being aware that this was the church where Hopkins had been assistant priest for a time. When I visited Balliol College, it was for tutorial lessons with my classics tutor, Mr. Dover, not for any sentimental reasons linking the college with Hopkins. The very air I gathered and released was as little associated in my mind with Hopkins as with Scotus. Nor, to tell the truth, did I much relish it, as it was so damp and depressing in the winter months, which lasted though the Michaelmas and Hilary terms.

All the same, it was perhaps during this time that I became better acquainted with the poems of Hopkins than I had been before. I attribute this acquaintance, however, not so much to any personal interest of mine as to certain Jesuit friends of mine, Francis Clark, Laurence Cantwell, and John Harriott, who did have such an interest in the poet. No doubt it was thanks to them that I dimly perceived the greatness of this Jesuit predecessor of mine in the Victorian age.

For my personal discovery of Hopkins and his poems, however, I had to wait till I came to Japan in 1954, after the completion of my undergraduate studies at Oxford. The occasion of this discovery I can date with some precision—to the July of 1956, when I went with other Jesuit students from our language school at Taura, near Yokosuka, to spend our summer vacation on the shores of Lake Kawaguchi, one of the five lakes at the foot of Mount Fuji. One day I went with a friend from Chicago, Tom Charbeneau, to a little headland overlooking the lake, with a fine view of Mount Fuji beyond. There we sat and tried to work out the meaning of that most difficult poem, "That Nature is a Heraclitean Fire". Tom had been taught literature, both the classics and English, in his American juniorate by Father Schoder; and it was he who chose this poem as a profitable form of mental exercise for us. In fact, it proved to be not just a mental exercise, but an enjoyable and exhilarating challenge, to puzzle out the sense of the seemingly meaningless words of Hopkins. From that headland I think I may say I returned a lover of Hopkins.

After that, however, I have no special memory of renewing my encounter with Hopkins, as I didn't have so many opportunities in any case. The rest of that summer I spent in distant Shimane Prefecture, teaching English to high-school students in the seaside town of Hamada; and the following January we completed our language course. Then I went on to study theology at our theologate to the west of Tokyo for the next four years. I was ordained priest in 1960, and once my fourth year of theology was over, I went to Hiroshima for my tertianship, or third year of Jesuit probation (the first two years having been spent in the noviceship). Of all this time I have no special Hopkinsian reminiscences.

It was only when I joined the faculty of English literature at Sophia University in 1962 that I began to pay serious attention to Hopkins. From the outset I was asked to teach his poetry at the graduate school, or perhaps it was I who chose to do so. Anyhow, I soon discovered that the best way of studying Hopkins, or any other poet, was to teach him, preferably in a small class of intelligent graduate students. First, we went patiently through "The Wreck of the Deutschland" stanza by stanza. It may have been the first time for me to read through that poem with anything like understanding. Then we went on to the sonnets of Hopkins. For each class I prepared printed material, based partly on comparison with Hopkins's other writings, partly on existing commentaries and books of criticism, partly on my own knowledge (from my Oxford years) and reflection. The outcome of all these efforts subsequently appeared in published form as *A Commentary on G. M. Hopkins' The Wreck of the Deutschland* and *A Commentary on the Sonnets of G. M. Hopkins*, published by the Hokuseido Press in 1968 and 1969, respectively.

It was in that same year, 1962, that I ventured to present a paper on Hopkins at the annual meeting of the English Literary Society of Japan then being held in Kyoto. The subject I chose was "The Underthought of Shakespeare in Hopkins", with special reference to the echoes of *King Lear* in the "terrible sonnets". One reason why I chose this subject was that I felt on stronger ground when relating Hopkins to Shakespeare, whose plays I had studied much more thoroughly than Hopkins's poems. For I still felt somewhat shaky about Hopkins, and I was afraid, when it came to question time, my ignorance would be exposed. To some extent my fears were justified when I found myself unable to give a satisfactory answer to a question raised by a Hopkins scholar, Professor Mifune Okumura, who from then onwards became a good friend of mine.

For the next ten years my study and teaching of Hopkins continued without event, apart from the publication of the above-mentioned commentaries. Then about 1970 the Hopkins Society was born. It was on the occasion of another meeting of the English Literary Society of Japan that another friend of mine, Mr. Kazuyoshi Enozawa, who had done his master's thesis on Hopkins's "The Windhover", introduced me to a friend of his, Professor Suekichi Omichi, as another Hopkins fan. Together we decided to go ahead with our combined interest in Hopkins, according to the Japanese motto *Sannin yoreba, Monju no chie*—"With three minds together, one has the wisdom of Monju" (the Chinese sage Mencius). So the Hopkins Society was formed; and the annual issues of the bulletin, *Hopkins Research*, began to appear the following year, with regular articles from my pen.

It was also from 1970 onwards that I began to organize summer tours of the British Isles for Japanese teachers and students. The second tour of 1972 was now planned in conjunction with the new Hopkins Society as a special Hopkins tour. After ten days for orientation at Canterbury, we went on tour round England, trying to fit in as many places of Hopkinsian interest as possible. Thus we visited Oxford and Stonyhurst, St. Beuno's and Holywell, Loch Lomond and Inversnaid, and above all Dublin, where we could see not only the former Jesuit house on St. Stephen's Green but also the cemetery of Glasnevin with the humble grave of Hopkins, shared by him with so many Irish Jesuits. On that occasion I was able to take many slides of places connected with Hopkins to show my students back in Japan, as it were following in the footsteps of Father Schoder, whose craziness in this respect I had now come to emulate, or rather to surpass.

In the following year, 1973, I was granted a sabbatical year from Sophia University, and I think I can claim to have spent it fruitfully. First, I went to Korea in February to spend a semester teaching at the Jesuit university of Sogang in Seoul. Then I went on to America for the summer, and there I took the opportunity of visiting Father Schoder himself at Loyola University, Chicago. From the time of his visit to Japan in the summer of 1964 we had cherished the idea of collaborating on an illustrated book on the poetry of Hopkins, for which he would provide the illustrations from his rich slide collection, while I would write the chapters on the basis of my commentaries. Now I was able to go through all his slides, including those of the front of St. Beuno's and of the sea at Harwich, and to select those which seemed most suitable for the book I had in mind—with one poem for each chapter and eight slides to illustrate each poem.

These slides I took with me on continuing my journey eastwards across the Atlantic to England in September. There in London I discussed our project with Anthony Wood, the editor for Paul Elek publishers, with whom I already had some contact in connection with a recent book on Chesterton. With his encouragement I went ahead with the manuscript of *Landscape and Inscape*, which I wrote in the space of three weeks during my stay in Cambridge in the Lent term of 1974 at the rectory of the Pugin church of Our Lady and the English Martyrs. Thus I could leave the finished manuscript and the slides with Anthony Wood before my return to Japan in March. The book itself came out in 1975, just in time for the unveiling of the Hopkins memorial in the Poets' Corner of Westminster Abbey that December, when it was conspicuously on sale in the Abbey Bookshop. The following year it received an award for the best illustrated book of the year from the Christian Publishers Association of America, where it had been jointly published by William Eerdmans of Grand Rapids, Michigan. Such an award was better deserved by Father Schoder than myself, since he had provided the illustrations; but it was certainly not deserved by the publisher, who, instead of distributing those illustrations in the text where they belonged, had gathered them together in groupings for the sake of economy—in spite of a generous grant obtained by Father Schoder. So instead of rejoicing over the publication with its subsequent award, I was left mourning over the ruin of my fond expectations.

(*Hopkins Research* 15, November 1986)

The Circling Bird

WHAT, I MAY ASK, was the favoured symbol of Hopkins as a poet? With which of all God's creatures did he prefer to associate himself? His answer may be found in one of the most impressive of his undergraduate poems, which opens with the haunting line, "Let me be to Thee as the circling bird" (dated 1865). Yes indeed. It is only natural for Hopkins, as a poet of both Nature and Grace, to compare himself, ideally speaking, to a bird, rising from earth to heaven on the wings of poetic inspiration.

Now let me ask a further question: With which among the many birds did Hopkins most readily identify himself? Such a precise identification is hardly to be found in his undergraduate poems. In them he makes occasional references to city pigeons, tower swallows, and rockdoves (in "The Alchemist in the City"), to eye-greeting doves and rooks (in "Myself unholy"), to nightingales and doves (in "The Nightingale"); but he names them merely as birds, without any sign of symbolism or self-identification.

It is only when we jump over the years of his "elected silence", from his undergraduate poems composed at Oxford to his more mature poems composed as a Jesuit student at St. Beuno's, that we find the poet identifying himself with a precise bird. Only, the identity of the bird changes from one poem to another, with a confusing yet charming variety, as providing us with one more instance of what he terms "pied beauty".

To begin with, from the moment Hopkins broke his seven years of self-imposed silence to write "The Wreck of the Deutschland", we find him identifying himself most readily with the dove, recalling the bird that had appeared most frequently by name in his earlier poems. He looks back to a certain moment of stress and strain in his past life—whether his conversion to the Catholic Church, or his vocation to the Society of Jesus, or his decision to compose this very poem. And then he solves his problem by whirling out wings of inspiration and flying "with a fling of the heart to the heart of the Host" (st.3). The thought is evidently inspired by the words of Psalm 54, "O that I had wings like a dove! For then I would fly away and be at rest." Then he goes on to congratulate himself on having been "dove-winged" and "carrier-witted"—with reference to carrier-pigeons.

Confirmation of this self-identification with the dove is to be found in two further poems. First, in "Hurrahing in Harvest" the poet again speaks of rearing "wings bold and bolder" and flying up to Christ, whom he professes to glean "down all that glory in the heavens". It is the same impulse of love that he has noticed in the dove. Secondly, in "The Handsome Heart" he recurs to the image of carrier-pigeons, with reference not only to the individual boy who chiefly figures in the poem but to all men, including himself. "What the heart is!" he exclaims, "which, like carriers let fly—/ Doff darkness, homing nature knows the rest."

But now, to return to the original mention of the "circling bird", how, we may ask, does this description apply to a dove or a pigeon? Is the poet thinking of the way a carrier-pigeon circles in the air on being released from its cage before sensing the right direction? Or may he not be thinking of another bird equally noted for its manner of circling in the air?

This question I ask in view of that other bird with which the name of Hopkins is chiefly associated in literary criticism, the feathered hero of "The Windhover". Here the image of circling in the air, even while hovering, seems to be suggested by the way the bird "rung upon the rein of a wimpling wing". At least, the note in the fourth edition of his *Poems* explains "to ring" as meaning "to rise in spirals". In this case, however, can we say that the poet is identifying himself with the bird? Isn't he rather contrasting himself with the bird? After all, the fact that he goes on to state, "my heart in hiding/ Stirred for a bird", seems to put a distance between the poet and the bird.

In one sense, of course, the contrast, with its implied admiration of the bird, may point to an ideal self-identification. Watching the falcon "in its riding/ Of the rolling level underneath him steady air", the poet feels an impulsive desire to be like the bird. It is the feeling we find also in Shelley, when he looks up at the skylark and compares it to "a poet hidden in the light of thought".

At the same time, however, it may be said that the whole point of the poem consists in a contrast not so much between the poet and the bird as between his foregoing envy of the bird in the octet and his subsequent submission of this feeling to Christ in the sestet. On the one hand, the poet recognizes that he can hardly hope to emulate the "brute beauty and valour and act" of the bird, least of all while he is engaged in the humdrum study of theology. On the other hand, he comforts himself—or rather it is Christ who comforts him—with the thought that by buckling to the service of Christ he can become, as chevalier or knight of Christ, "a billion times told lovelier, more dangerous" than the bird.

In another sense, moreover, one may suspect a hidden identification between the poet and the bird, not so much in the bird described in the poem as in the bird he may have been watching at St. Beuno's College. I mean the stuffed bird in a glass cage which was actually at St. Beuno's in Hopkins's time, as part of the Waterton Collection and which bears the significant caption, "The Kestrel or Windhover". Thus one may imagine the poet meditating one morning on "The Kingdom of Christ", as given by St. Ignatius in his *Spiritual Exercises*, while standing in front of this stuffed bird. In the bird he may well have recognized a likeness with himself in his life of abstract study at St. Beuno's. But then, soaring upwards on the wings of a poetical and spiritual inspiration, he may have "caught" imaginative sight of the free bird in all its "brute beauty and valour and act". And so the contrast he goes on to draw between the bird and himself is that between himself as he would like to be and himself as he is now.

In this poem the heart of the poet stirs for one kind of bird, the windhover. But in other poems he experiences a similar stirring for other kinds of bird. Such, for example, is the skylark in "The Caged Skylark", where we find much the same kind of contrast as that which I have suggested in "The Windhover". For there is an obvious parallel between the stuffed bird and the "skylark scanted in a dull cage" and between the hovering bird in "the big wind" and the "daregale skylark" amid its "free fells". The poet is also thinking of himself both in the stuffed bird and in the caged bird; and so he goes on to draw a contrast between himself in his weary studies and the skylark in its native freedom. For the time being he is spending life "in drudgery, day-labouring-out life's age"; but he longs to follow his "mounting spirit", according to his hope of rising with Christ at the last day.

In identifying himself, therefore, as "the circling bird", Hopkins, it appears, saw himself in a variety of birds, in the dove, the windhover, and the skylark. At the same time, in his opening words, "Let me be to Thee", he seems to be thinking not only of himself but also of God. His desire for himself is to be like a bird, following the direction of his "mounting spirit" as a poet. But in his later poems we find him identifying God himself in terms of a bird. So in this early poem may we not listen to his words as echoed by God, "Let Me be to thee as the circling bird"?

Certainly, in his later, Jesuit poems we find God repeatedly represented in terms of a bird, especially a mother bird brooding over the eggs in her nest and protecting them from harm. This is the image implicit in the two references to divine feathers in "The Wreck of the Deutschland", even if for the sake of tradition and alliteration the poet speaks of God as "Father". Thus in stanza 12 he exclaims, "O Father, not under thy feathers"; and again in stanza 31 he admires the "feathery delicacy" of God's "lovely felicitous Providence". Again, in "God's Grandeur" he envisages the Holy Ghost brooding over the bent world "with warm breast and with ah! bright wings". And that is why, in his poetic opinion, "there lives the dearest freshness deep down things".

This image of a mother bird covering her "bevy of eggs", or her "nested cluster of bugle blue eggs thin", recurs in two other poems, "In the Valley of the Elwy" and "The May Magnificat". In the latter poem the bird is precisely identified as a song-thrush, or throstle, who is sitting on her "bugle blue eggs". This in turn looks back to the earlier sonnet on "Spring", with its juxtaposition of "thrush's eggs" that "look little low heavens" and the song of the thrush "through the echoing timber".

For Hopkins, as in certain strands of Christian tradition, God is both father and mother. But he also recognizes this divine attribute of motherhood as bestowed in overflowing measure on the Virgin Mary. In "The May Magnificat" he hails her as "the mighty mother", with an implication of the ancient earth goddess, and he sees her as "sympathizing/ With that world of good,/ Nature's motherhood". Also in "The Blessed Virgin compared to the Air we Breathe" he goes on to compare the motherly providence of Mary to "Wild air, world-mothering air,/ Nestling me everywhere".

All this, of course, has reference to birds in general; and if Hopkins speaks particularly of the thrush, it may have been because he had in mind Browning's famous "Home Thoughts from Abroad", with its mention of "the wise thrush". Or it may have been because of his fondness for the "bugle blue eggs" of the thrush.

In another poem, however, his curtal sonnet on "Peace", Hopkins recurs to his favourite image of the dove, which he here names "wild wooddove". This time he mentions the cooing of the bird only to draw attention to its brooding over its nest. At the same time, he implicitly recalls the traditional identification of the Holy Spirit as a dove, brooding over the waters of creation (in Genesis 1) and of "the Yore-flood" (in Genesis 8), as well as over the waters of the Jordan at the baptism of Jesus. For in the form of a dove the Holy Spirit is presented as the Spirit of Peace.

Now, therefore, putting all these bird images together, we find in Hopkins's poems a basic identification of both himself and God in terms of a bird, preferably but by no means exclusively a dove. In his present actuality, the poet may have felt himself more like a stuffed or a caged bird;

but in his "mounting spirit" he longs for his native freedom to soar up into the air and to circle "high there" with the windhover. At the same time, while envisaging this ideal self in terms of a bird, soaring and singing in the sky, he looks up to God as both father and mother, extending arms like wings over the bent world. He also looks up to the Virgin Mary as she shares the motherly attribute of God, and he rejoices in the vision of "all things rising, all things sizing" in the world.

In conclusion, we may say that for Hopkins, as for Newman who received him into the Catholic Church, there were "two luminous beings", himself and God, and that, more specifically than Newman, he conceives these two beings as birds of light—all birds in general, but the dove in particular.

(*Hopkins Research* 16, August 1987)

The Place of Hopkins in Poetic Tradition

EVER SINCE T. S. Eliot published his essay on "Tradition and the Individual Talent" in 1919, we have become accustomed to thinking and speaking of individual poets in relation to some larger tradition. The further idea of "placing" writers, both poets and novelists, has similarly been emphasized ever since F. R. Leavis published his book on *The Great Tradition* in 1948, in which the author's indebtedness to Eliot is undeniable. Yet long before the time of both Eliot and Leavis, Hopkins was writing in much the same vein, notably in his long letter to Canon Dixon from Roehampton on December 1/16, 1881.

In this letter Hopkins is primarily speaking of Dixon's poems, which he places in what he calls "the school of the prae-Raphaelites"[*sic*]; and he goes on to trace a line of literary descent from "this modern medieval school" to "the Romantic school . . . of Keats, Leigh Hunt, Hood, indeed of Scott early in the century". He further derives this school of Keats from "that Elizabethan tradition of Shakespeare and his contemporaries which died out in such men as Herbert and Herrick". In the same letter, he draws another contrast between the Romantic school and "that of the Lake poets and also of Shelley and Landor", adding that the latter seem to him to represent "the mean or standard of English style and diction, which culminated in Milton". One particular difference he notes between the two schools is that, whereas the former are "great realists and observers of nature", the latter are "faithful but not rich observers of nature". All this Hopkins says in connection with the poems of Dixon, but reading between the lines we may recognize a reflection on his own poetry. This leads us to ask to which of the two schools Hopkins sees himself as belonging; or in other words, which of the two seems to have his preference. To begin with, considering his praise for the Romantic school of Keats, for its realism and observation of nature, and his own excellence in this regard, we may well place the poems of Hopkins in the line of that poetic tradition which reaches back through Keats, and maybe Tennyson, to Shakespeare and so to the Catholic Middle Ages.

This supposition seems to be confirmed by Hopkins's frequent praise in his letters for the poetry of both Keats and Tennyson, not to mention Shakespeare. From his own early poems, as exemplified in "A Vision of Mermaids", he is said by his friend Bridges to "betray the influence of Keats", even if in his later poems he is seen to have outgrown that influence. And towards the end of his life, in two of his letters written from Dublin to Coventry Patmore, he vigorously defends what he calls the masculine quality of Keats's genius, for all his admitted sensuality, which at times amounts to "an unmanly and enervating luxury" (May 6, 1886). He also draws a comparison between Keats's poems, which were after all "only the work of his first youth", and "Shakespeare's early work" (Oct. 20/24, 1887)—implying that, if Keats had lived, he might even have come to rival the great Shakespeare.

As for Tennyson, Hopkins sees in his poetry "a mean or compromise between Keats and the medievalists on the one hand and Wordsworth and the Lake School on the other". From the first, he was no less in love with Tennyson than with Keats; but on September 10/11, writing to his friend Baillie, Hopkins speaks of "a horrible thing" that has recently happened, namely, "I have begun to doubt Tennyson." This doubt is based on what he now perceives as a vein of "Parnassian" language pervading the poems of Tennyson, namely, that language which "is spoken on and from the level of the poet's mind, not . . . when the inspiration which is the gift of genius raises him above himself". Much of Tennyson he has now come to see as typically Parnassian, whereas if Shakespeare rarely palls, it is because "he uses . . . so little Parnassian". All the same, Hopkins remains an admirer of Tennyson, regarding him (as he tells Dixon in a letter of Feb. 27/Mar. 13, 1879) as "one of our greatest poets", whose "poetry appears 'chryselephantine', always of precious mental material and each verse a work of art."

On the other hand, in contrast to his continuing admiration for Keats and Tennyson, Hopkins seems to have had little respect for Wordsworth. In his above-mentioned "Parnassian" letter, he gives it as his personal opinion that this is "because he writes such an intolerable deal of Parnassian". Nor was he, in Hopkins's opinion, such a rich observer of nature. Still, in all his large poetic output there is one notable exception that Hopkins is more than willing to admit; and that is the great ode on "Intimations of Immortality". Of this poem he writes to Dixon (Oct. 1886) that it "seems to me better than anything else I know of Wordsworth's, so much as to equal or outweigh everything else he wrote". He even regards it as expressing one of those rare moments in which, as he says, "human nature . . . saw something, got a shock", and has been "in a tremble ever since". As for himself, too, he confesses, "I am, ever since I knew the ode, in that tremble." He is even prepared to propose the fanciful patriotic opinion that "St. George and St. Thomas of Canterbury wore roses in heaven for England's sake on the day that ode, not without their intercession, was penned."

What Hopkins says here about the "Immortality" ode seems almost enough to entice him away from the Keats-Shakespeare medieval tradition and to align him with the Wordsworth-Milton classical tradition. This new alignment may seem strengthened by the fact that he himself regarded his poetic masterpiece, "The Wreck of the Deutschland", as a Pindaric ode, belonging to that ode tradition which reached back through Wordsworth's ode and Milton's "Lycidas" to the classical odes of Pindar in ancient Greece. In particular, he comments with undisguised delight on how in this ode "the rhymes are so musically interlaced, the rhythms so happily succeed (surely it is a magical change, 'O joy that in our embers'), the diction throughout is charged and steeped in beauty and yearning (what a stroke, 'The moon doth with delight'!)." Thus it looks as if we can say that the prosody of Wordsworth, at least in the case of this ode, had a profound impact not only on the mind but also on the poetic practice of Hopkins.

Yet another quality Hopkins shares not so much with Keats and Shakespeare as with Wordsworth and Milton is the prophetic idea of poetic inspiration. This is what he seems to imply in the opening stanza of "The Wreck", where he acknowledges, "Over again I feel thy finger and find thee." Not that he ever, like Wordsworth and Milton, claims a prophetic or even priestly function in his poetry, but, unlike them, he is in fact a priest writing poetry, and he may be said to have had a priestly purpose in all his poetry, as it were mediating the presence of Christ in the world of nature to the minds of his readers. He did indeed speak of his poems, in a letter to Bridges of February 15, 1879, as a distraction from his priestly activities: "I cannot in conscience spend time on poetry." Yet when he came to compose them, he could hardly do so save as a priest, and even as a prophet. It may even have been the presence of this impulse in him, or his resistance to this impulse, that precipitated his period of "dark sonnets" in Dublin, in between "Spelt from Sibyl's Leaves" and "That Nature is a Heraclitean Fire and of the comfort of the Resurrection".

In not a few of his letters, moreover, we find Hopkins engaged in a determined effort to imitate Milton rather than Shakespeare. His very idea of sprung rhythm in "The Wreck" was partly suggested to his mind by that counterpoint rhythm of which he sees Milton as the "great master", especially in "the choruses of *Samson Agonistes*" (Author's Preface). The verse of Milton he elsewhere compares, in a letter to Dixon (Oct. 5, 1878), to Purcell's music, as "something necessary and eternal"; and he remarks how incomparable is the art of Milton, "ahead of his own time as well as aftertimes in verse structure"—just as, we may add, Hopkins's own verse was ahead of his Victorian age. He also confides to Bridges his hope "to have a more balanced and Miltonic style" (Feb. 15, 1879)—a hope he thought he had to some extent realized in his sonnet "Andromeda", in which he endeavoured (as he tells Bridges on Aug. 14 of that year) "at a more Miltonic plainness and severity than I have anywhere else".

If Hopkins's Miltonic style is to be judged by a poem such as "Andromeda", however, it can hardly be said to have brought out the best in his poetic talent. Rather, to quote the words of Browning in "Rabbi Ben Ezra", "the best is yet to be" in the "dark sonnets", which may well be regarded as the outcome of the poet's Jacob-like encounter with the angel of prophecy. In that case, we may well turn back from the influence of Milton and Wordsworth (for all their prophetic claims) to that of Shakespeare and Keats. For it is in these later sonnets, together with the fragments from "St. Winefred's Well", that the influence of Shakespeare (rather than Keats) comes to prevail over the poet's mind. Not that he ever sets out to imitate Shakespeare (apart from the speech of Caradoc) as he did with Milton; but he has always seen Shakespeare, at least from the time he said so in his early letter to Baillie (Sept. 10/11, 1864) as "utterly the greatest of poets".

In conclusion, it may be said that Hopkins, even more than Tennyson, bestrides both traditions, while inclining rather to Keats than to Wordsworth, rather to Shakespeare than to Milton, and rather to the Catholic Middle Ages than to the pagan classics. It may further be added that there is yet a third school on which he comments in the above-mentioned letter to Dixon, namely, the modern or sentimental school, of which the prime example is for him Lord Byron. Of this school, however, he has little good to say, except that it has "a deep feeling"; otherwise it has "the most untrustworthy and barbarous eye for nature, a diction markedly modern, and their keepings any gaud or a lot of Oriental rubbish". And there, without more ado, he drops it.

(*Hopkins Research* 17, August 1988)

The Message
of Hopkins

AMONG MODERN literary critics the word "message", particularly with the addition or implication of "moral", is hardly a fashionable one. So to speak of "the message", let alone "the moral message", of Hopkins would appear to be inviting derision. "Art," it is dogmatically proclaimed, "contains no message: the artist is no preacher: he merely expresses his personal vision in his particular medium: he isn't trying to persuade, to convince, to convert, still less to brain-wash anyone: he is no proselytiser, no propagandist: he is just an artist."

Such is the all too common idea of art, including poetic art, among modern critics. But when we consider the poetic art of Hopkins, we have to take into account not only what modern critics say, with all their modern presuppositions and prejudices, but also what Hopkins himself as poet intended in his poetic composition. Did Hopkins himself, we may ask, have a message, even a moral message, in his poetry? Did he intend to say something to his readers, something he regarded as important, even urgent, in his poetry? Was it his aim, as best he could, to persuade his readers to accept what he saw as good, and to dissuade them from falling into what he saw as evil?

In answering this question, we have to remember that Hopkins was a Jesuit, a very traditional kind of Jesuit, deeply imbued with the spirit of his founder, St. Ignatius Loyola. And it is, I dare affirm, impossible to be such a Jesuit without having a message, an urgent moral and spiritual message, for others. For the aim of a Jesuit, inspired by the fiery idealism of St. Ignatius, is nothing short of winning the whole world for Christ, according to the desire which that saint puts into the mouth of Christ in his meditation on the Kingdom. Any time a Jesuit spends in the pursuit of any other, worldly aim is nothing but a waste of time.

True, Hopkins himself felt, and expressed, certain misgivings regarding his pursuit of poetry, as being not altogether consonant with his religious and priestly vocation. To break his long poetic silence, which he had imposed on himself—no one else had imposed it on him—from the time of his entrance into the Society of Jesus, he required more than the mere permission, he desired the positive suggestion, if not the explicit command, of his superior. So it was only when the rector of St. Beuno's College expressed the desire that someone should compose a poem on the subject that Hopkins took him at his word and set about composing his Pindaric ode on the shipwreck of the *Deutschland*, as his first poem of significance after having become a Jesuit.

Then, we may ask, is there a moral message in this poem? May we say that Hopkins is preaching a kind of poetic sermon to his readers? If so, what is it that he wants to say to us? How does he want to improve us?

First, I would say there is most definitely a moral message in "The Wreck of the Deutschland". The poet is most certainly seeking to persuade and convert his readers to Christ, in pursuance of that ideal of the Kingdom of Christ which he has made his own in the course of seven long years in the school of St. Ignatius. It may not be presented in the customary form of a sermon, beginning with the customary words, "My dear brethren", after the declaration of the text; but it certainly aims at producing the effect of a sermon in persuading, even converting the hearers, or readers—though the effect depends not just on the poet's aim but also on the disposition and response of the readers.

Then again, what is this message? It may be stated, quite simply, in the opening words of the Gospel of Jesus Christ, where he himself seems to be doing no more than echoing the refrain of St. John the Baptist, "Repent, for the kingdom of heaven is nigh."

Where does Hopkins say this? He doesn't say it in so many words, but it is what remains at the back of his mind throughout this poem. What he shows is, above all, what he takes the tall nun as seeing in the shipwreck amid the stormy weather. "She that weather sees one thing, one", namely, the coming of Christ "in the storm of his strides" to save her and all her fellow passengers, and implicitly all readers of the poem, thereby "royally proclaiming his own" so as to bring them safely to the kingdom of his Father in heaven.

This is, however, to put everything in a nutshell and to present what I see as Hopkins's conclusion before having given all the evidence. So now let me return to the beginning and spell out the poetic and homiletic message of the poet in detail.

From first to last, it is true, we don't find the poet addressing his readers in the way we expect a preacher to address his congregation. He is rather raising his mind and heart to God in a prayer of praise, beginning with the solemn invocation, "Thou mastering me, God!" and culminating in two magnificent doxologies in the last stanzas of the two parts of the poem. In this respect, the poem is to be seen as more of a meditation than a sermon, one that is addressed not to the people but to God, one that is inspired by the meditations in the *Spiritual Exercises* of St. Ignatius. In any case, I am not saying that Hopkins means to offer a poetic sermon or a kind of didactic poem in "The Wreck of the Deutschland". All I say is that in this poem he has an urgent moral message to convey to his readers, even when addressing his words not so much to them as to God. After all, if it had been his intention to pray to God, while meditating on the shipwreck, he might as well have prayed in silence, while meditating in silence. For God has no need of man's words, since he looks into the heart of man. So if Hopkins avails himself of poetic words to express his meditation on the shipwreck, it isn't so much for God's sake as for his readers', for the purpose of bringing those readers closer to God and thus of bringing the kingdom of God closer to its realization on earth.

This aim the poet, in fact, presents at the end of each of the doxologies with which he concludes the two parts of his poem. At the end of the first part he prays with urgent insistence, "Make mercy in all of us, out of us all/ Mastery, but be adored, but be adored King"—where everything leads up to his final stress on "King". Then at the end of the second part he specifies the object of his prayer more precisely as the new life of conversion, "Now burn, new born to the world"; and he goes on to pray earnestly for "our King" to come "back, Oh, upon English souls!"

This is the poet's principal aim, as well in his poem as in his whole life as a Jesuit, nothing less that the conversion of England to Christ. Not that he limits his desire of conversion to the English; but it is to them that he primarily addresses his words, in the English language in which he writes his poem. What he desires in the first place is the extension of Christ's kingdom among his fellow countrymen, according to the prayer recited at Benediction "for the conversion of England". Nor is this a prayer he offers somewhat vaguely to Christ; but it is his hope that this poem may contribute to the answering of his prayer, insofar as his readers are influenced by his words.

Further, what the poet prays at the beginning and the end of his poem may be seen as an elaborate extension of the cry of the tall nun, who is the heroine of the poem. All she says, as the poet records in stanza 24, is, "O Christ, Christ, come quickly." It seems to be no more than a simple prayer to Christ for speedy salvation from the waters of affliction; but the prayer, and the desired salvation, are not for herself alone. As the poet has already stated in stanza 19, the nun not only "rears herself to divine/ Ears", but her call also rises up "to the men in the tops and the tackle" for all "the storm's brawling". In this way she brings comfort—or rather, through her breast as bell, it is "lovely-felicitous Providence" that brings comfort—to "the comfortless unconfessed of them". So in this way the shipwreck is turned into "a harvest", and the tempest carries the human grain for the heavenly barn.

This is what the poet has described in vivid detail in the second part of the poem, the part he composed first in point of time before going on to the prefatory first part. It is evidently what had inspired him in his previous reading of the newspaper accounts of the shipwreck, as it had distinguished this particular shipwreck in his mind from the other accounts of shipwreck he would have read in newspapers about this time. It is also what he insists on in his description of the event in the second part, where he leads up to "the call of the tall nun" and inquires precisely, "What did she mean?"

Here some readers may well form the impression that the poet wastes a lot of time offering one suggestion after another as to the nun's meaning, before rejecting them one after another. In much the same way, he may seem to have wasted a lot of time introducing the tall nun and her sisters in the preceding four stanzas. It is as if he is just padding out the poem. Yet it all serves to build up to the climax in which he sees, as with the nun's eyes, a vision of Christ walking to her over the waters, as Christ had been seen by his disciples walking to them over the waters of Genesareth. Then so great is his excitement that he seems quite at a loss for words, though his very loss is a poetic gain: "But how shall I . . . make me room there:/ Reach me a . . . Fancy, come faster—/ Strike you the sight of it? Look at it loom there,/ Thing that she . . . There then, the Master."

Here we may notice that the poet is not only at a loss for words, but his excitement and bewilderment and stuttering inadequacy last only so long as he sees "it" as a "thing", or impersonal apparition, something that comes gliding over the waters like a ghost. Once, however, he recognizes it as not just a thing but a person, the person of Christ himself, he changes his tone from one of almost frenzied excitement to one of intense satisfaction, from one of incoherence to one of calm recognition. "There then! the Master,/ *Ipse*, the only one, Christ, King, Head."

In other words, here precisely is the "one thing, one" which the tall nun has seen in "that weather". Here is the "one fetch" which she is said to have in her. It is what the poet has already indicated, without identifying it, in stanza 19. Now at last, after an interposition of eight stanzas, he is out with it, identifying it in stanza 28 as "the only one". Thus he keeps up an effective feeling of suspense, so as to make the final outcome (in Shakespeare's words) "the more delayed, delighted".

This isn't just what the poet presents in his poem for the entertainment or the aesthetic appreciation of his readers.

Rather, he is doing his utmost to involve them in the same experience, if only vicariously by means of the imagination. So they, too, may come to share with him, in a Christian version of Aristotle's *catharsis*, in the nun's vision of Christ. In this respect, his method may be regarded as a kind of pedagogy, or mystagogy, leading his readers as initiates to a sacred mystery. Indeed, he describes the incident as a mystery in the precise, etymological meaning of the word, as a sacred ceremony serving to reveal the inner meaning of death as a gateway to eternal life. Nor is this only a mystery in the ancient Greek sense of the Eleusinian mysteries, but also in the applied Christian sense by which we are taught to look through the death of Christ to his resurrection and that of all those who believe in him.

In this context we may the more easily appreciate the point and purpose of the more theological and personal first part of the poem. In the first ten stanzas the poet seems to be rambling here and there, recalling events from his past life and from the life of Christ, before finally getting down to what we have been expecting from his title to be the main object of the poem, the wreck of the German ship. This is because in the first part he wishes to place this particular incident in its wider context, in relation both to himself as poet and to Christ as inspirer of the poem.

To be precise, the poet is recalling how in his past life he has experienced a kind of shipwreck, a death followed by a new life of conversion; and he is reflecting how this moment looks back to the time of Christ, to the "day/ Of his going in Galilee", culminating in "The dense and the driven Passion". Nor does this apply to himself alone, a perception of what he made his own in the moment of his conversion to Christ. It applies no less to all men, whether Christians or not, inasmuch as Christ has come to save all men by means of his death on the cross. This is what Hopkins states at the climax of this first part, just before coming to his first doxology: "Hither then, last or first,/ To hero of Calvary, Christ's feet—/ Never ask if meaning it, wanting it, warned of it—men go."

This is the universal truth of Christ and Christian salvation which Hopkins proposes, by way of preface or prelude to his account of the shipwreck which follows in the second part. He looks from himself to Christ, and from a moment of strain and stress to a succeeding moment of relaxation, so as to prepare his readers to enter all the more deeply into the experience and to see all the more clearly the vision of the tall nun, as first she is wrecked with all the other passengers and then she sees Christ coming over the waters to save her. Then finally, with a word or a cry, she communicates—and the poet in her also communicates—her vision to all who may hear her and so receive the grace of salvation.

In this the poet isn't just preaching to his readers, as a second-rate preacher might do in a sermon, implying a separation between himself and them—with himself standing on a pulpit elevated above them, while they are seated passively in the pews below. Rather, he aims at involving them, first in his own past experience, then in the nun's present, parallel experience, and lastly in the archetypal experience of Christ in his passion and death on the cross and his resurrection from the dead.

This is a purpose which the poet realizes more effectively by directing his words in prayer to God than in exhortation to his readers. It is also for this purpose that I am speaking not of any exhortation in the poem, since such exhortation is usually made on a conscious level, but of a "moral message", since such a message is best conveyed at a subconscious level, by leading the hearers or readers away from themselves and their petty concerns to a higher, purer, more divine view of human life.

Thus, if I may repeat what I have been saying again and again, what the nun sees in her dying moments and declares by her cry to her fellow passengers, the poet goes on to declare to his readers by means of the poem. Thus his aim, like the nun's in her dying moments, and Christ's on the cross as saviour and inspirer of the poem, is the coming of the kingdom of Christ into the hearts of his readers. Lastly, I may add, this is also the aim of a Jesuit critic, as he sets out to interpret the aim of the Jesuit poet, as he originally intended his poem to be understood, according to the motto of the founder of the Society of Jesus, *"Ad Majorem Dei Gloriam"*—To the greater glory of God.

(*Hopkins Research* 18, June 1989)

Hopkins and the Oxford Movement

   THE OXFORD MOVEMENT, to begin with, may be defined as a movement of renewal within the Anglican Church arising out of the more widespread movement of political and educational reform in the western world. In England the latter movement was sponsored by the newly emerging Liberal party under the leadership of Lord John Russell, but the aim of Newman and his friends in the Anglican Church was by no means similar to that of Lord Russell and his friends in the Liberal party. Rather, in the Liberals Newman and his friends saw a serious threat to the very existence of both Church and State in England. They saw that what Russell was advocating as a Liberal, or what had till then been called a Whig, was a secularist separation of Church and State, which was in turn a triumph for the Protestant "faction" in the Church of England. On the contrary, what Newman and his friends emphasized was the need of returning to the Catholic ideal of tradition, according to the teaching of the Caroline divines in the seventeenth century and the earlier Fathers of the Church, such as Athanasius and Augustine, but without what they regarded as the accretions and corruptions of the Roman Church.

This movement had its beginnings, as Newman later recalled them in his *Apologia pro Vita Sua*, at Oriel College, Oxford, where Newman was himself a fellow from 1822 and a tutor from 1826, and from within which he received his appointment as vicar of St. Mary's university church in 1828. After an impressive tour of Italy and Sicily with his friend Hurrell Froude in 1832–33, during which he composed his famous hymn, "Lead, kindly Light", he returned to England to find the country filled with excitement over the political reforms proposed by the Liberals. His own concern and that of his friends was voiced at this time in the celebrated sermon preached in St. Mary's church by an elder member of their group, John Keble, on "The National Apostasy". In it the preacher inveighed against the liberalism and secularism of the age, and from then onwards it was regarded by Newman himself as the starting point of their movement.

The true leader of the movement, however, wasn't Keble, though it was he who set the ball rolling, but Newman from his central position as vicar of St. Mary's at the heart of the religious life of Oxford University, as that university may be seen in turn as the heart of the Church of England. From now on Newman initiated two series of statements or publications giving expression to the ongoing ideas of the movement. First, there was the series of "Tracts for the Times", composed by himself and his friends under his editorship, in which they drew attention to various aspects of the Catholic "faction" in the Church of England, thereby earning for themselves the nickname of "Tractarians". These tracts were subsequently published in book form under the title of *Via Media*. They culminated in Tract 90 in 1841, in which Newman proposed a Catholic interpretation of the Thirty-Nine Articles of the Anglican Church, drawn up under Protestant influence in the beginning of Elizabeth's reign, only to find his position publicly repudiated by both his Church and his university.

Meanwhile, Newman had also been giving a series of inspiring sermons at St. Mary's church from Sunday to Sunday, stating not the more polemic positions of the tracts but the devotional ideal behind them, notably the ideal of the guiding light of God's presence and providence. It was this idealism that appealed to the minds of his university audience, far more than the polemics of the tracts; and one of Newman's many devoted followers, Matthew Arnold, spoke for his contemporaries in his oft-quoted reminiscence of the sermons: "Who could resist the charm of that spiritual apparition, gliding in the dim afternoon light through the aisles of St. Mary's, rising into the pulpit, and then, in the most entrancing of voices, breaking the silence with words and thoughts which were a religious music—subtle, sweet and mournful? Happy the man who in that susceptible season of youth hears such voices! They are a possession to him forever."

When the turning point came, with the official rejection of Tract 90, Newman had no other option than to resign his living at St. Mary's and to retire into seclusion with his friends at Littlemore outside Oxford. There, as he reflected on his religious position, he found himself steadily moving from the Anglican to the Roman Catholic position in view of his favourite idea of "development"— the idea that not all Christian doctrine is to be found explicitly stated in the Bible (as the Protestants maintained), but that much is left implicit for further development within the Church. This was the idea he had found fully stated by St. Vincent of Lerins as early as the fifth century, in his "Commonitorium":

It is desirable that development should take place, and that there should be a great and vigorous growth in the understanding, knowledge and wisdom of every individual as well as of all the people, on the part of each member as well as of the whole Church, gradually over the generations and the ages. But it must be growth within the limits of its own nature, that is to say, within the framework of the same dogma and of the same meaning.

Such were the thoughts Newman went on to present in his own *Essay on the Development of Christian Doctrine*, which he published shortly after his formal submission to the Church of Rome in 1845.

He then made his way to Rome to study for the Catholic priesthood; and there he was ordained as early as 1847. He then sought admittance into the Congregation of the Oratory, which had been founded by St. Philip Neri, a close friend of St. Ignatius, in the sixteenth century. Returning to England, he established the first Oratory at Birmingham; and that remained the base of his operations from then till the end of his life—apart from that period of frustration in the mid-fifties when he was occupied with his attempt to found a new Catholic university in Dublin. It was after his return from Dublin to Birmingham that he was drawn into another controversy with the novelist Charles Kingsley. The latter had accused him of insincerity in his conversion to Rome; and so Newman was prompted to present "the history of his religious opinions", centring on the Oxford Movement, under the title of *Apologia pro Vita Sua* in 1864.

Meanwhile, Newman's departure from Oxford University and the Anglican Church had not spelt the end of the Oxford, or Tractarian, Movement; but it continued at Oxford under Newman's senior friend at Oriel College, Edward Bouverie Pusey, who subsequently became canon of Christ Church. It was from now on, in connection with Pusey and with his other Anglican friend Henry Liddon, that we find a young undergraduate student from Balliol College, Gerard Manley Hopkins, drawn with other young friends of his into the movement. Only it was the stronger influence of Newman, particularly on the occasion of the publication of his *Apologia*, that led Hopkins in turn to follow him into the Church of Rome in 1866.

Brought up as he was within a devout Anglican family in Hampstead and educated at a strongly Anglican school in Highgate, it seemed only natural for Hopkins, on joining Balliol College at Oxford, to be drawn into the continuing Oxford Movement, under the aegis of both Pusey and Liddon. It was about the time that Pusey had been making the sensational charge of heresy against the Regius Professor of Greek, Benjamin Jowett, who was soon to become Hopkins's tutor and subsequently master of Balliol. It was a year later that Newman published his *Apologia*, which served to revive the main issues of the Oxford Movement that had led to his conversion to Rome. Hopkins found himself increasingly persuaded by Newman's reasons—reasons that were by no means merely aesthetic (as some recent critics have maintained) but almost coldly logical. As he himself wrote in a letter of 1866 to Liddon, "I can hardly believe anyone ever became a Catholic because two and two make four more fully than I have." What he meant by two and two making four he explained in a letter to his father at the same time, announcing his forthcoming reception into the Catholic Church:

> I am surprised you should say fancy and aesthetic taste have led me to my present state of mind: these would be better satisfied in the Church of England, for bad taste is always meeting one in the accessories of Catholicism. My conversion is due to the following reasons . . . (i) simply

and strictly drawn arguments partly my own, partly otherwise, (ii) common sense, (iii) reading the Bible, especially the Holy Gospels, where texts like 'Thou art Peter' . . . (iv) an increasing knowledge of the Catholic system . . . which only wants to be known in order to be loved.

It was already on July 17 that he wrote in his diary: "It was this night . . . that I saw clearly the impossibility of staying in the Church of England." But it wasn't till October 21 that he made his formal submission to the Church of Rome, in the presence of Father Newman at the Birmingham Oratory.

This movement of Hopkins from the Church of England to that of Rome is reflected in several of his poems composed about this time and recorded in his diary. Thus in October 1865, after a note indicating the possibility, "If ever I should leave the English Church", we come upon two significant poems illustrating not just the possibility but also the probability. One of them, untitled, begins with the words, "Let me be to Thee as the circling bird." In the course of the poem Hopkins states his longing for "a changeless note" and "the authentic cadence", which, he says, he has "discovered late"—which must be the infallible teaching of the Roman Church, though he doesn't explicitly say so. As for the other poem, its very title, "The Half-way House", echoes a passage from Newman's *Apologia*: "There are but two alternatives, the way to Rome and the way to Atheism. Anglicanism is the half-way house on the one side, and Liberalism is the half-way house on the other." In this poem, moreover, Hopkins refers to the Anglican Church as "my national old Egyptian reed", in punning contrast to the "cross-barred rod or rood" of Rome; and he adds that only in the latter can he take "love's proper food", the Eucharist, "in the breaking of bread".

The following year Hopkins wrote a poem for Lent entitled "Nondum", or "Not yet", implying that the time for his formal submission to Rome hadn't yet come. Much of the poem is devoted to thoughts of darkness and despair, with echoes not only of Tennyson's "In Memoriam" and Arnold's "Dover Beach", but also of Newman's "Lead, kindly Light" (as contrasted with "the encircling gloom") and that passage in the *Apologia* where the author looks "Out of myself into the world of men, and there I see a sight which fills me with unspeakable distress". Only in the end of his poem does Hopkins turn to a glimpse of hope: "Then, to behold Thee as Thou art,/ I'll wait till morn eternal breaks." And that is also the end of Newman's hymn: "And with the morn those angel faces smile/ Which I have loved long since, and lost awhile." That morning dawned on Hopkins on October 21, 1866, when he went north to Birmingham and was formally received by Newman into the Catholic Church. He went on to follow Newman not into the Oratory of St. Philip, but as a teacher at the Oratory School founded by Newman, before entering the noviceship of the Society of Jesus at Manresa House, Roehampton, to the southwest of London, in 1868.

Now we may pause and consider the question, What was the influence of the Oxford Movement and his conversion to Rome on Hopkins's later Jesuit poetry, composed after his seven-year period of "elected silence", from "The Wreck of the Deutschland" onwards? It is, in fact, to be found already at the beginning of that great poem of his, which may be called a poem of conversion, though seemingly devoted to a tragedy of shipwreck. It is precisely the experience described so impressively in the second stanza, beginning with the words, "I did say yes/ O at lightning and lashed rod", and continuing with detailed reference to "the walls, altar and hour and night" when this happened to him. That it was a real experience, we have Hopkins's own word for it in a letter to his friend Robert Bridges, though when it occurred he doesn't say. Still, it isn't unlikely that it was the night when, as he records in his diary for July 17, 1866, "I saw clearly the impossibility of staying in the Church of England"—or perhaps a moment before, which seems to be echoed in "Nondum", with its epigraph from Isaiah, "Verily, Thou art a God that hidest Thyself"—or even before, in the poem beginning with the words "My prayers must meet a brazen heaven", where the poet feels himself "battling with God".

This is also the experience Hopkins later recalls in one of his terrible sonnets, entitled "Carrion Comfort". There, too, he recalls "that night, that year/ Of now done darkness I wretch lay wrestling with (my God!) my God". In "The Wreck of the Deutschland", however, he goes on to recall how he managed to escape from his horror, when he "fled with a fling of the heart to the heart of the Host". That is to say, he encountered the love of God in the holy Eucharist, which is exactly how he concludes his poem "The Half-way House", with the words of Eucharistic invitation: "You have your wish; enter these walls, one said:/ He is with you in the breaking of bread." Similarly, in the aftermath of the terrible sonnets, we come upon the sudden ending of the darkness of death in "That Nature is a Heraclitean Fire", when with another "fling of the heart" the poet cries, "Enough! The Resurrection,/ A heart's clarion!" This time, however, he finds his joyful outcome not so much in "the breaking of bread" as in the reality of heaven, to which the sacrament points with its sacred symbolism. For after having composed the sonnet on July 26, 1888, the poet passed to his eternal reward on June 8, 1889—within a year.

This may bring us back to the idea of rebirth or renaissance in Hopkins, inasmuch as, with St. Paul, he sees his conversion in terms of death to his old self and renewal in Christ. This is how he concludes "The Wreck", as being the most autobiographical of his poems, first with reference to the resurrection of Christ: "Now burn, new born to the world,/ Double-natured name,/ The heaven-flung, heart-fleshed, maiden-furled/ Miracle in-Mary-of-flame", and secondly, with extended reference to others, especially his poor fellow countrymen, for whom he prays that "Our King (may come) back, Oh, upon English souls!" and "Let him easter in us, be a dayspring to the dimness of us, be a crimson-cresseted east,/ More brightening her, rare-dear Britain, as his reign rolls."

Similarly, at the end of his other wreck poem, "The Loss of the Eurydice", Hopkins prays earnestly for "My people and born own nation,/ Fast foundering own generation." This is indeed the apostolic ideal at the heart of his poetic and priestly energy, as he strives to convey to others that vision of divine love which he has found for himself and made his own, from the time of those early poems, as when he ends "Let me be to Thee as the circling bird" with the strong desire, "Love, O my God, to call Thee Love and Love." In the same vein, in "The Half-way House" he prays, "Love, come down to me if Thy name be Love." Such was the prayer which was granted to the poet both at his conversion in Oxford and Birmingham and at his death in Dublin. And now, like the five nuns whose memory he celebrates in "The Wreck", and no doubt like Newman himself, who went before him in conversion but followed him a year later in death, we may think of Hopkins, too, as having attained "the heaven-haven of the reward", where he is in a position to remember "us in the roads" and to pray for us as a saint in heaven.

(*Hopkins Research* 19, August 1990)

Hopkins and the Spirit of Man

In 1916, in the midst of World War I, Robert Bridges, poet laureate since 1913, brought out his well-known anthology entitled *The Spirit of Man*. In its subtitle it was described as "An Anthology in English and French from the Philosophers & Poets made by the Poet Laureate in 1915 & dedicated by gracious permission to His Majesty The King". In his preface the compiler speaks of "a special purpose" he had in mind in his compilation of the book, for which he professes to provide "a sufficient guide . . . in the page-headings". The contents are an idiosyncratic mixture of English and French, prose and poetry, while the authors of the selected passages and the precise sources are relegated to notes at the end of the book, so as not to distract the reader's attention from the passages themselves. As for their arrangement, it is neither logical nor chronological, but based on a free, personal association of ideas evidently arising out of the serious world situation, ideas whose interconnection is indicated in the headings of each page. The general theme, implied in the title of the book, is, as the compiler states in his preface, "that spirituality is the basis and foundation of human life", that "man is a spiritual being, and the proper work of his mind is to interpret the world according to his higher nature, and to conquer the material aspects of the world so as to bring them into subjection to the spirit."

Of special interest to students of Hopkins is that this anthology not only is compiled by the poet's lifelong friend and confidant—not to mention critic—but also includes as many as six poems by Hopkins, of which three are here printed for the first time; whereas "Spring and Fall" (No. 9), "The Candle Indoors" (No. 269), and "The Habit of Perfection" (No. 385) had already appeared in Alfred Miller's third volume of *The Poets and the Poetry of the Century* (1893). Not that six poems from one poet is particularly deserving of note, considering how many passages there are from Shakespeare and Milton, Wordsworth and Coleridge, Keats and Shelley, as well as from the friends of both Bridges and Hopkins, Canon Dixon (no fewer than fifteen) and Digby Dolben (also six). All the same, what is unique about the passages from Hopkins, in contrast with other passages, is that so many of them are printed here for the first time from manuscripts in the possession of Bridges himself. Considering, too, that this anthology was published only two years before Bridges brought out his edition of Hopkins's *Poems* for the Oxford University Press in 1918, it looks as if he was putting out feelers in the form of these six poems, partly to test the reactions of the reading public, partly to anticipate his intended publication of all the poems in his possession.

As for the six poems of Hopkins included in this anthology, apart from the three mentioned above they are: the first stanza of "The Wreck of the Deutschland" (No. 53), "In the Valley of the Elwy" (No. 358), and "The Handsome Heart" (No. 369). Considered as a selection of Hopkins's poems, this group may well strike us as a surprising one, seeing how few of them have turned out to be among Hopkins's most popular poems and how many more popular ones of his have been passed over. In the context of the anthology, however, we have to remember it was Bridges's purpose not to anthologise Hopkins or the other poets represented in his selection, but to illustrate his own developing thoughts and moods from various poets and authors, including Hopkins. Thus, in the light of the above-mentioned page headings, "Spring and Fall" comes under the caption of "Sorrow's Springs", the first stanza of "The Wreck" under that of "Worship", "The Candle Indoors" under that of "Conscience", "In the Valley of the Elwy" under that of "Hospitality", "The Handsome Heart" under that of "Pupil & Teacher", and "The Habit of Perfection" under that of "Self-Renunciation".

Further, considering these six poems in view of Hopkins's correspondence with Bridges, and the latter's continual complaint of obscurity in his friend's poems, one might assume that Bridges would have included only those poems he considered easier for the common reader to understand—such poems as "Spring and Fall", written to an imaginary little girl, no doubt in order to avoid the criticism of obscurity, and "The Habit of Perfection", which is the only poem in the anthology belonging to Hopkins's undergraduate years with Bridges at Oxford. As for "The Handsome Heart", it had evidently been a favourite poem of Bridges's from the beginning, though Hopkins himself says he "thought it not very good" (Aug. 14, 1879). The first stanza of "The Wreck", which Bridges famously called "the dragon at the gate" of his friend's poems, may have been included partly for its intrinsic impressiveness, partly to prepare the minds of readers for the subsequent publication of the whole poem. What is more, whereas in Hopkins's letters to Bridges we get the impression of an obtuse, even infidel friend, in this admittedly sparse selection of his poems we see the depth of Hopkins's long-term influence on his friend's mind; and that may well have come to a climax with the contemporary catastrophe of World War I. In the anthology as a whole we see the compiler turning to religious and Christian sources of spiritual comfort in a world at war; and for this change of heart one may suspect he was in no small measure indebted to his old Jesuit friend.

Now we may come to a consideration of how these six poems fit into the context and main purpose of the anthology. First, it has to be noted that *The Spirit of Man* is divided into four books, which have no titles beyond the aggregation of their page headings. Thus Book I opens with the theme of "Dissatisfaction" (no doubt with a world at war), and so the compiler comes to "Sorrow's Springs", the heading for "Spring and Fall". This thought leads his mind upwards from his feelings of deep distress on earth to the "Idea of God" and "Spiritual Love & Praise", and so to "Worship" as the heading for the first stanza of "The Wreck". In the second book there is nothing of Hopkins, as the compiler dwells on the romantic ideas of "Beauty" and "Ideal Love", "Childhood" and "Nature". But as he turns to the further ideas of "Sorrow" and "Sin", "Ethics" and "Philosophies" in Book III, the thought of "Conscience" moves him to choose Hopkins's sonnet "The Candle Indoors"—that strange poem in which the poet suddenly turns from a mild mood of regret for others to a savage criticism of himself. Finally, it is in Book IV, which deals with "Christian Virtue" and "Social Virtue", that we come upon most of the poems from Hopkins.

First, the sonnet "In the Valley of the Elwy", though admittedly " far-fetched" (in the words of the poet, quoted by the compiler in his end notes), is offered as an example of "Hospitality", in connection with the virtues of "Loving-kindness" and "Sympathy". Secondly, "The Handsome Heart" comes under the heading of "Pupil & Teacher" in a series of personal poems that follow on the theme of "Commiseration"; and here, too, one sees the compiler's mind moving upwards from those who suffer on earth to the "Saints in Heaven". It is this movement which further reminds him of his friend's undergraduate poem "The Habit of Perfection", and he inserts it under the heading of "Self-Renunciation". From now on the compiler proceeds to illustrate such themes as "The Master's Will", "Sanctification for Life", "The Fight against Evil", and "The Happy Warrior". In them he seems to turn his eyes once more to the war going on around him, but now he sees it in terms not just of the daily newspaper but of the Church militant on earth, as she toils towards "The Heavenly Kingdom" and "The True Light".

From all this we may draw the conclusion that the function of Hopkins in this movement of "The Spirit of Man", small and insignificant though it may seem in terms of mere quantity, is the all-important one of spiritual guide, or *psychopompos*, to his friend Bridges—a function not unlike that of Virgil to Dante in the *Divina Commedia*, as his heavenly escort from the depths of the *Inferno* through the stages of the *Purgatorio* to the beginning of the *Paradiso*. Only, once they reach this point, it is Bridges, not Hopkins, who can go no farther but can only look up "in a glass darkly" to the heavenly vision.

(*Hopkins Research* 20, August 1991)

Hopkins as Ecological Prophet

❧ "POETS," PROCLAIMED SHELLEY, "are the unacknowledged legislators of the world." Poor Shelley! How little he knew of the real world! How few of this world's legislators over the few centuries since he uttered those words have paid any attention to his ambitious claims! How few of them have even acknowledged him as one of their number! Yet if not as legislator, at least as prophet, the poet may be granted his due of acknowledgment. As for Shelley himself, I am not so sure. His spirit soared too high above the clouds for his feet to be planted on the earth; and that is an indispensable condition for all would-be legislators. As for his Victorian successor, Gerard Manley Hopkins, however, I have no doubt. Events in the past decade or so have amply secured his right to be regarded as a prophet and champion of the environment, of world ecology, of Mother Earth.

In the poems of his Jesuit maturity, from his years at St. Beuno's College onwards, we notice Hopkins's continuing and developing concern for man's natural environment, as he sees it increasingly threatened by the ongoing Industrial Revolution. "Generations have trod, have trod, have trod," he complains in "God's Grandeur", "And all is seared with trade, bleared, smeared with toil." Elsewhere, in "The Sea and the Skylark", in contrast to those two natural noises "too old to end", he cries shame on "this shallow and frail town" of Rhyl, sunk as it is in "sordid, turbid time" and draining fast, as if with the outgoing tide, "towards man's first slime". Even in his dear university town of Oxford, with its many memories of Duns Scotus, he notes with indignation the "graceless growth" of its "base and brickish skirt" around the new railway station, which has confounded the "rural keeping" of "folk, flocks, and flowers".

Above all in "Ribblesdale" the poet's indignation is directed against "dear and dogged man", who is "to his own selfbent so bound, so tied to his turn". This man he relates in particular to the industrialists, who are so wedded to themselves and their ideas of selfish, financial profit, so unconcerned or even reckless about the good of the earth on which they are standing and from which they derive their own well-being. They are so ready "To thriftless reave both our rich round world bare/ And none reck of world after", whether in another world or in a future generation of this world. Indeed, what the poet saw in his own time, over a hundred years ago, may he not also be said to have foreseen of our time, when the blind greed of those industrialists in Victorian England has borne its bitter fruit, not only in England with her notorious "black country", but all over the world? So now we see the world's politicians, journalists, and environmentalists gathered at Rio de Janeiro, shaking their heads at the appalling excesses of modern industry and scientific progress, while seeking even at this eleventh hour to devise means of evading the all but imminent destruction of the planet.

Still, if Hopkins may be regarded as a prophet of doom and ecological destruction a hundred years ahead of his time, he isn't only that. No true prophet can be content with the utterance of mere warnings or threats of disaster. It is his mission, as we see in the case of Jeremiah, not just to root out, pull down and destroy, but also to build up and plant new life. As for Hopkins, while he saw the industrialists of his time intent on building factories and apartments for their underpaid workers, with railways for the convenient transport of their products, as well as of passengers, what could the poet and prophet do with his wild and whirling words but, as the other prophet Isaiah warns, bring forth wind? Well, we may point to the hidden meaning in his words, as it were the "winged seeds" borne by the "wild West wind" celebrated by Shelley. For a long time they may "lie cold and low, each like a corpse within its grave", yet as winter turns to spring, they will come to fill "with living hues and odours plain and hill". So now, as the world's environmentalists gather at Rio with "brows of such care, care and dear concern", we find the eminence of Hopkins acknowledged—in this aftermath of the centenary celebrations of his lonely death in Dublin—more than ever before.

What, then, is this poet's prophetic message to the world at this critical moment for our future? It is a message not of doom or destruction, but of hope and new life. As he continues in "God's Grandeur", "And for all this, nature is never spent", since "There lives the dearest freshness deep down things." Yet how, we may wonder, can he give expression to such overweening confidence? Or how can we echo his words of confidence, when we see how much worse, even to the extent of desperation, the world has become in our time? Simply because, as he goes on to say, "the Holy Ghost over the bent/ World broods with warm breast and with ah! bright wings". Here is a faith in divine providence that runs like a golden thread through all Hopkins's poems, in abrupt contrast to that other, leaden thread of despair over "what man has made of man", in poetic counterpoint and creative tension.

At the same time, beside this Christian faith in God—in the providence of the Father and his "feathers", in the presence of the Son with "his world-wielding shoulder", and in the brooding of the Holy Ghost "with warm breast and with ah! bright wings"—there is in all Hopkins's poems a basic teaching of love that is expressed not so much in precept as in example, not so much in deed as in suffering and lament. Whereas the motivation behind the world's representatives gathered at Rio de Janeiro for the security of the environment and the salvation of the planet seems to be little more than an enlightened self-interest, Hopkins insists, not without a sob in his voice, on the need of loving Earth for her own sake. Thus, with his imaginary child named Margaret, he grieves "over Goldengrove unleaving", recognizing in the falling leaves reflections of "the things of man". Similarly, in his own adult person, while following in the footsteps of the pre-Romantic William Cowper, he bewails the felling of his "aspens dear", the poplars growing along the river bank at Binsey, and man's unfeeling destruction of their "sweet especial scene", their "rural scene". Above all, to return to "Ribblesdale", he addresses Earth herself as "sweet Earth, sweet landscape", with blatant disregard for what many Victorians from Ruskin onwards decried as "pathetic fallacy", yet with deeper, humanly instinctive personification.

Indeed, for Hopkins, as both poet and prophet, everything may be seen as coming to a point in this personification of Earth as (in Shakespeare's words) "Nature's mother"; and all his poetry may be seen as coming to a point in this one poem. It makes him sound indeed like a forerunner of modern environmentalism, in presenting Earth as appealing to heaven "with no tongue to plead, no heart to feel", but with only her silent being. As for that, he charmingly adds, "Thou canst but be, but that thou well dost", since, he reflects, "what is Earth's eye, tongue, or heart else, where/ Else, but in dear and dogged man?" And where, we may add, is Earth's eye, tongue, and heart more eloquently expressed than in this poem, in which Hopkins so stands out in his and our time as prophet and champion of the planet Earth?

(*Hopkins Research* 21, August 1992)

This-ness in Hopkins

It was during his study of philosophy at St. Mary's Hall, Stonyhurst, that Hopkins first came upon "Scotus on the Sentences", that is, the commentary of Duns Scotus on the "Sentences" of Peter Lombard, "and was flush", as he records in his journal for August 3, 1872, "with a new stroke of enthusiasm". Then what was it, we may ask, that so impressed the mind of Hopkins with the seemingly arid logic-chopping of Duns Scotus? Not, surely, the logical manner of verbal expression, but some meaning implicit in the words, something unique or "arch-especial" in the philosophy of Scotus.

There is, for instance, the way Scotus championed the thesis of the Immaculate Conception of the Virgin Mary, even against so redoubtable an adversary as St. Thomas Aquinas. And so, as Hopkins went on to recall in his sonnet on "Duns Scotus's Oxford", the latter "fired France for Mary without spot". There is also the emphasis Scotus lays on the infinity no less than on the unity of the divine essence; and this may have provided Hopkins with a precious clue to the paradox indicated in "Pied Beauty", that "All things" on earth, with all their dappled variety and unique individuality, "He fathers forth whose beauty is past change." There is also the way Scotus traces his theology of the Incarnation not just back to the "day of his going in Galilee", or even to the decree of Redemption following on the Fall of Man, but to the very foundation of the world. For this reason it is that the poet can recognize the presence of "our Saviour" both in the "glory of the heavens" and in "the azurous hung hills" in "Hurrahing in Harvest".

No, I would say, echoing the words of Hopkins himself from "The Wreck", "but it was not these" aspects of the subtle doctor's thought that chiefly impressed the poet's mind, but Scotus's characteristic theory of this-ness, or *haecceitas*, which is punningly identified in the spelling of mediaeval Latin with *ecceitas*, from *ecce*, meaning "Look!" or "Behold!" This may remind us of Hopkins's other poem "The Starlight Night", with its opening exclamation, "Look at the stars! Look, look up at the skies!/ O look at all the firefolk sitting in the air!" There is something altogether childlike in such excited enthusiasm, recalling as it does a particular incident during the poet's life at Stonyhurst, as recorded in his journal for August 17, 1874: "As we drove home the stars came out thick: I leant back to look at them."

In this poem Hopkins sums up all the beauty of the stars as "*this* piece-bright paling", the lovely barn or fence that "shuts the spouse Christ home". He implies the same thing in his other poem "Hurrahing in Harvest", where he also exclaims, concerning "all that glory in the heavens", "*These* things, *these* things were here and but the beholder/ Wanting." Here the immediate reference may be to the "lovely behaviour of silk-sack clouds" in the daytime; but the implication is of Milton's words in *Paradise Lost* Book IV, where Adam asks the angel, "But wherefore all night long shine *these*, for whom/ *This* glorious sight, when sleep hath shut all eyes?" Yes, it is surely the beauty of such a starry night that raised the mind and heart of Hopkins heavenwards in delighted enthusiasm, even the enthusiasm with which he had become flush on his first encounter with "Scotus on the Sentences" in the Baddely Library at Stonyhurst. Amid the infinite variety and multitude of all the stars the poet recognized a uniqueness and a unity to which, with Scotus, he readily assigned the quality of *haecceitas*.

This is an enthusiasm, or ecstasy, that draws the poet as it were out of himself in an impulsive desire to leap upwards. It is the impulse we find in stanza 5 of "The Wreck", when the poet seems to "kiss my hand/ To the stars, lovely-asunder/ Starlight, wafting him out of it". Here, it is true, we find no use of "this", but only its rhyme-word "kiss". But sure enough, in the next stanza, we do meet "this"—"(and few know this)"—in conjunction with its other rhyme-word "bliss".

Here let me dwell for a moment on these two rhyme-words for "this"; for they are not without significance to the poet's sensitive ear. First, in "The May Magnificat", "this", coming at the end of the line, "Well, but there was more than *this*", serves to introduce "Spring's universal bliss". Then, in case the foregoing "this" may have seemed too weak in comparison with the "bliss" that follows, the poet goes on to sum up everything in springtime with "*This* ecstasy all through mothering earth". For him there is indeed ecstasy in "this". There is a similar contrast between the weaker "this" and the ecstasy that follows in "God's Grandeur", where the poet sums up the weariness of trade and toil, with the smudge and smell of man, in the phrase, "And for all *this*," only to raise his eyes to "the brown brink eastward". There in the light of the rising sun he sees "the Holy Ghost" as a mother bird brooding "over the bent world . . . with warm breast and with ah! bright wings".

Here we find no precise mention of ecstasy, for all its evident implication. But we may catch a clearer glimpse of it in what is surely the most ecstatic of Hopkins's poems, "The Windhover". From the outset the ideal of *haecceitas* is present in "I caught *this* morning". Again, as at the end of "God's Grandeur", it is the morning, only here its uniqueness or "this-ness" is emphasized. And again, the poet is lost in ecstasy at the sight of a bird. Up above, he beholds the bird "in his ecstasy"; while down below, "my heart in hiding/ Stirred for a bird."

Then, what about the other rhyme-word with "this", namely "bliss"? There is one other instance among Hopkins's major poems in which all three rhyme-words are grouped significantly together, in "The Soldier". They occur in alternate lines in the sestet, when we are shown Christ first in heaven, where he "bides in bliss", next leaning down from heaven, to fall on man's neck with a "kiss", and finally exclaiming at the man's noble deed, "Were I to come o'er again . . . it should be *this*." Thus, from "bliss" through "kiss" we come to the climax of "this", than which there is (for Hopkins) nothing greater.

This is a climax. But what, we may ask, is a climax if it isn't followed by an anti-climax? At least, that is the case with Hopkins and his poetry. His bright sonnets are inevitably followed by dark sonnets, not without the company of a very subdued "this". It is almost ironical, the way his favourite "this" follows him as it were into exile, with an altered demeanour. Thus in the first of his dark sonnets, "Carrion Comfort", he typically mourns over "*these* last strands of man in me". It is as if the singularity of "this" has become dissipated into the plural of "these", as he feels (like the earth in "Spelt from Sibyl's Leaves") his dapple at an end, "astray or aswarm, all throughter, in throngs". Then, in the darkest of the dark sonnets, "I wake and feel", he sums up his sad sights and ways with a rueful "this"—while adding that it isn't even unique to himself but spoken "with witness". As for himself, after uttering all these laments, he goes on to make the sad confession, "I see/ The lost are like *this*". Then, too, in his further sonnet on "Patience", after speaking of "war" and "wounds", the weariness of "times" and "tasks", the lot "To do without, take tosses, and obey", he observes, "Rare patience roots in *these*, and *these* away,/ Nowhere." Thus he moves from the sad singular of "this" to the sadder plural of "these".

Even when the poet seems to have recovered from his sadness in "That Nature is a Heraclitean Fire", there is no more ecstatic "this", but only the humble reference to himself as "*This* Jack, joke, poor potsherd, patch, matchwood", if in association with "immortal diamond". Such is the humility echoed again in "The shepherd's brow" in more general terms, as "Man Jack the man is, just". Only in his last sonnet, "To R. B.", does Hopkins seem to recapture something of his former delight in "this-ness", even while paradoxically lamenting its absence. "Sweet fire the sire of muse," he confesses, "my soul needs *this*." But then, after speaking of "this" as a need, not a possession, he proceeds to the other, weaker rhyme-word "miss", as a verb whose object is "The roll, the rise, the carol, the creation". Yet even from such a "winter world" he can raise his eyes and his mind to the further rhyme-word of "that bliss", as at least a memory of past splendour.

In thus following the fortunes of "this-ness", as the central idea of Hopkins's Scotism, through his major poems—and there are many more that might have been mentioned—it may appear that there is no need, after all, to make a choice between this and other ideas I mentioned at the beginning of this essay. Rather, once I enter into this one idea of "this-ness", I find the others clustering round it in the way that "birds of a feather flock together". It is, for instance, intimately related to the above-mentioned identity of infinity and unity in God, which Hopkins shows more generally in "Pied Beauty" and more specifically in Christ in "As kingfishers catch fire". "For Christ," he says, "plays in ten thousand places,/ Lovely in limbs, and lovely in eyes not his/ To the Father through the features of men's faces." It inculcates that in Christ as Son in the eyes of his Father the just at once retain their human individuality, or "this-ness", and show forth their corporate unity.

Further, with a little of that ingenuity or subtlety for which Scotus was famous in his time, one might go on to show how this vision of the universal Christ both in the world and in men, especially in the just, is linked with the doctrine of the Incarnation, as having taken place from the foundation of the world. And this in turn may be connected with the Scotist defence of the Immaculate Conception, placing Our Lady by the side of Our Lord from the beginning. Thus in his long poem on "The Blessed Virgin compared to the Air we Breathe", Hopkins looks to the universality of the Virgin Mary, not only, as in "The May Magnificat", in the revival of nature in springtime, but also in the blue sky as manifesting the universality of her chosen colour. "Yea," he says, "mark you *this*"; and he goes on to speak of "*this* blue heaven", which matches the green of nature on earth, and "*this* bath of blue", which serves to slake the fire of the sun.

It isn't therefore surprising, to return to the sonnet on "Duns Scotus's Oxford", if in his memory of that great mediaeval philosopher in his Oxford setting Hopkins comes to a climax of "this-ness", before leading on to the fire with which he filled France "for Mary without spot". For as he comes to his sestet, he feels as if he is breathing in the marsh air of the university with a kind of ecstasy, as he exclaims, "Yet ah! *this* air I gather and I release/ He lived on; *these* weeds and waters, these walls are what/ He haunted who of all men most sways my spirits to peace."

(*Hopkins Research* 23, December 1994)

Hopkins and the Renaissance of Rhythm

Between Hopkins's undergraduate poetry and that which emerges in 1876, when he at last broke his "elected silence", there is a great difference. It is all the difference, one might say, between the minor and the major religious poet. His "self-denying ordinance" in destroying his early poems on entering the Jesuit noviceship in 1868, or what he himself later regretted as a "massacre of the innocents", was immensely fruitful in the long run. From that time onwards, instead of composing poems, he kept a journal of detailed observations of nature; and that provided him with rich material he could go on to use in his subsequent poetry. At the same time, he kept his ear open to the various sounds of nature and human speech, of the Hebrew psalms and Greek lyric verse, of Old English metre and even Welsh poetry (when he took up the study of Welsh on going to St. Beuno's College in North Wales for his study of theology in 1874).

All this time, from 1868 onwards, as he later recalled in a letter to his friend Canon Dixon, he had "haunting my ear the echo of a new rhythm which I now realized on paper". The occasion was the shipwreck of a German ship named the *Deutschland*, at the mouth of the Thames in December

1875, with five Franciscan nuns among the two hundred people on board. The ship had been bound for America; and the nuns, who had been driven from their homeland in Germany on account of certain anti-Catholic laws, were among the seventy-eight victims drowned. Hopkins also recalled how he was "affected by the account" and how, when he mentioned his reaction to the rector of the College, Fr. James Jones, the latter "said that he wished someone would write a poem on the subject". This was the hint which Hopkins welcomed as absolving him from his self-imposed resolution of poetic silence. So he set to work on his great poem which he entitled "The Wreck of the Deutschland".

This is a poem not just about what it seems to say, the shipwreck of the *Deutschland* with the consequent drowning of the five nuns, but also about the metaphorical shipwreck that had taken place in the poet's own life on the occasion of his conversion to the Catholic Church in 1866 and his subsequent vocation to the Society of Jesus, which he entered in 1868. It was a shipwreck of his human attachments to his family in London, to his Church at Oxford, to his ties with many Anglican friends, to his intellectual promise and his poetic ambitions. So what he saw in the experience of the drowning nuns, as depicted in the second part of his poem, he had already undergone in his own experience, as depicted in the preceding Part I.

The outcome was a truly revolutionary poem in the history of English literature. It may be said that there has been nothing like it either before or since, though it may possibly be compared with the subsequent "Hound of Heaven", also a poem of conversion, by Francis Thompson, and with T. S. Eliot's "Ash Wednesday". In its time, however, it was a completely new kind of poem, and so it could never be published in its time, not even by Hopkins's fellow Jesuits, when he submitted "The Wreck" for publication in the Jesuit journal *The Month*. It was certainly too revolutionary for Victorian readers, inured though they were to theories of both political and biological revolution.

What, then, was so new about the poem? Almost everything, it may be answered. The idea of the poem, the form of poetic diction, the vocabulary and grammar, the use of stress and alliteration and, above all, the rhythm incorporating all these qualities in one—not the conventional rhythm characterized by Hopkins as "running rhythm" but a new "sprung rhythm" of his own devising, which he felt obliged to explain to his readers in an "Author's Preface". Needless to say, as Hopkins admits in this preface, his new rhythm wasn't entirely new. It was already to be found in several nursery rhymes, such as "Ding, dong, bell", in Old English alliterative poems such as *Piers Plowman*, in Milton's choruses to *Samson Agonistes*, even in common speech. In particular, he points to the pervading influence of a Welsh form of poetry called *cynganedd*. But what is new in Hopkins's poem is the way he uses this rhythm in conjunction with rhyme, alliteration, and assonance, in an altogether unique mode of expression. For him the rhythm is the best means of conveying to his readers his deep feeling of enthusiasm at what he calls the "inscape" and "instress" of nature.

Here let me pause for a moment on these two characteristic coinages of Hopkins, used as they are in close connection with "sprung rhythm". They first appear in notes written by him for his tutor at Oxford on the thought of the pre-Socratic philosopher Parmenides. They are also frequently found in his subsequent diaries, expressing various aspects of his observations of nature. "Instress" refers to the inner activity in the world of nature, proceeding from the original inspiration of the Holy Spirit; while the outcome of that creativity is seen in the many forms of "inscape", or inner aspects of landscape. The more Hopkins tries to recapture his glimpses of "inscape" in nature, the more he responds to the power of "instress", and this is what he conveys to his readers in the "sprung rhythm" of his poetry. From the opening stanza of this new poem, we are impressed by something unique in its rhythm, with its strong, steady beat indicative of firm faith in God: "Thou mastering me/ God, giver of breath and bread." Such is the rocklike faith with which he goes on to interpret the seemingly disastrous event of the shipwreck. Yet the emphasis here isn't so much on "God", which remains significantly unstressed, as on the personal relationship between God and himself, "Thou . . . me", and again, at the end of the stanza, "Over again I feel thy finger and find thee." In it we may recognize an echo of Newman's "two luminous beings", himself and God—except that Hopkins puts God first, as well as last, as he goes on to close the last line with the sprung rhythm of "find thee".

Again in the second stanza we may detect the continuing influence of Newman, as the poet turns from his assertion of faith in God to the "encircling gloom" of the world around him. Here the world is for him more than mere gloom: it is the snowstorm, with thunder and lightning, the "lightning and lashed rod" of a more than natural terror. So whereas Newman (in his *Apologia*) could only lament over the gloom of the surrounding world cut off from God, Hopkins declares, more positively recognizing a meaning in the gloom, "I did say yes/ O at lightning and lashed rod."

Here the imagery of a storm seems to point to the snowstorm in which the German ship was wrecked at the mouth of the Thames. But here the poet is speaking not of the nuns or other passengers on board, but of himself, discerning a parallel in his own life, possibly the moment of his conversion. Then it was that in a moment of stress and strain, when he seemed to be wrestling with God himself, he "did say yes"; and then in all that stress and strain he found the creativity of God and the inspiration of the Holy Spirit, as he felt his "midriff astrain with, laced with fire of stress".

Thus "The Wreck of the Deutschland" is much more than a ballad describing in swiftly moving terms the tragedy of a shipwreck, or an elegy on the tragic deaths of the five nuns followed by an expression of hope in their resurrection. It is also an intensely personal poem, recalling a moment of intense stress in the poet's own life, the stress of conflict in wrestling with a personal problem, behind which he comes to see the hand of God. Then what he has found in himself he goes on to project into the experience of the five nuns in the disastrous setting of shipwreck. Or rather, it is on the occasion of that experience that he recalls what has happened in his past life. And out of all this, as he perceives in it the creative activity of God, he acquires a new poetic creativity of his own amid the peculiar stress of sprung rhythm. So within himself he looks from his personal limitations to the eternal tension within the heart of God, or what he calls "the stress of selving" in God. And so within his poetic theory and practice is implied a whole theology of stress which is altogether unique in Christian literature.

The particular problem Hopkins goes on to deal with in the second part of his poem, with precise reference to the shipwreck, is that of innocent suffering as seen in the case of the five nuns, who have been sent into exile from their fatherland by unjust laws. Their fate is shown in the light of the poet's faith—analogous to Newman's—in divine providence, which is present and operative in all things in order to bring them all to a happy outcome. This faith is once again presented in rocklike terms, as directed to him who is "ground of being and granite of it, past all/ Grasp God". And God is in turn shown as "throned behind/ Death". Such rocklike faith we find once again uttered with the insistent beat of sprung rhythm, in a series of stressed monosyllables with hardly an unstressed syllable in between. What is more, this is no blind faith, such as that postulated by the Danish Protestant philosopher Søren Kierkegaard, but a faith that borders on vision, when the poet identifies himself with the nuns and through their eyes sees Christ himself coming to them through the storm, walking over the waters of the North Sea, as before he had walked over the waters of the Sea of Genesareth.

From now on Hopkins felt no more need to revert to his former "elected silence", but he continued his composition of poems with sprung rhythm—if in such moments as his delicate conscience would allow him by way of respite from his main priestly work. For this purpose he now found that the form of poetry most suited to his poetic genius and his priestly circumstances was the sonnet, which offered him a challenge and a means of concentrating his mind within a narrow compass. So from his pen we now have a series of "bright sonnets", expressing a mood of optimism and enthusiasm in faith that triumphs over all worldly obstacles.

Among these poems special attention may be paid to that which the poet came to regard as "the best thing I ever wrote", namely, "The Windhover". The poem is dated May 1877, about a year after the completion of "The Wreck of the Deutschland", while the poet was still engaged in his theological studies at St. Beuno's College. It is the poem in which he supremely expresses his ideas of inscape and instress in the world of nature, while finding within it the deep message of Christ to his heart. In particular, he expresses his ideas in the concrete image of a bird, a kestrel, hovering high up in the sky, while at the same time he hears the voice of Christ speaking to him in his heart and using the flight of the bird as a parable.

Once again, from the outset of the poem one is impressed by the poet's magnificent use of sprung rhythm: "I caught this morning morning's minion, king-/ dom of daylight's dauphin, dapple-dawn-drawn Falcon." Here the words are all intimately woven together by alliteration and assonance, in a majestic rhythm leading up to a climax of enthusiasm: "How he rung upon the rein of a wimpling wing/ In his ecstasy! Then off, off, forth on swing." Once again, too, we come upon a series of stressed monosyllables with hardly an unstressed syllable in between, expressive of almost breathless admiration at what the poet goes on to hail as "the achieve of, the mastery of the thing".

There is, however, much more to the poem than just the poet's enthusiasm at the inscape and instress of the bird in flight, which is all contained within the octet. More important to the poet is the lesson he learns from this experience through the words of Christ spoken to his heart. What Christ, as king speaking to his knight, has to teach him is a warning not to rest in this created, mortal, brute beauty, which soon passes away, but to look through it to "God's better beauty, grace" in submission and obedience. For in all this natural beauty, whether in oneself or in others, there is the danger of pride, or of envy. Only when the poet, as "chevalier" of Christ, buckles down to the Jesuit rule in humble obedience, then "the fire that breaks" from him becomes "a billion times told lovelier" than the brute beauty of the windhover. Under this rule he may have to endure a life of poverty and suffering, the way of the cross; but then he is compared to the "blue-bleak embers" of a fire that "fall, gall themselves, and gash gold-vermilion". That is to say, as he has said of the nuns in "The Wreck", he will come by way of death with Christ on the cross "To bathe in his fall-gold mercies, to breathe in his all-fire glances".

Here again we may see how Hopkins's renaissance of rhythm is at one with his renaissance of religion, or his conversion to Christ. As in "The Wreck", so now in "The Windhover", the poet is evidently reliving his memory of conversion, as reproduced for him through the *Spiritual Exercises* of St. Ignatius, which may be described as a textbook for conversion. In particular, among these exercises of special significance for an understanding of "The Windhover" is that on "The Kingdom", in which Christ is shown as king making an appeal to his knightly followers. In this poem the lordly Falcon is described as "dauphin", or crown prince, of the kingdom of daylight; but Christ, as king of heaven and earth, addresses the poet as his knight or "chevalier". Later on, Hopkins added the subtitle "To Christ our Lord", as if to emphasize the relevance of the meditation to his poem.

Further, it has to be noted that religious conversion is never once for all but remains an ongoing process, following certain well-defined stages. Traditionally, three main stages have been distinguished, those of affirmation, negation, and excellence, which are also known as three "ways". The first is a way of delight at finding, in the first flush of conversion, how all things point to God and look (as poets say) "from nature to nature's God". The second, however, is a way of desolation on finding how God is, it seems after all, absent from all things, with nature no longer a help but a hindrance to devotion.

Such is the contrast we may recognize in the poetic development of Hopkins, from his earlier "bright" sonnets to his later "dark sonnets". The former he composed in the aftermath of "The Wreck", especially during his last year of theological studies at St. Beuno's College and for a few years after. But the latter he went on to compose in his land of exile, in Dublin, whither he was sent in 1884 as professor of Greek at the newly revived Royal University. There he was following once more in the footsteps of Newman, not only in teaching at the university originally founded by Newman, but also in experiencing there a frustration analogous to that of Newman, a frustration which at times made him feel as if he were going mad.

It was in this land of exile "among strangers" that Hopkins experienced what St. John of the Cross famously termed "the dark night of the soul"; and this experience he went on to describe in a series of sonnets, mostly written in 1885, that are among the darkest and most terrible poems in the English language. Now he no longer feels any enthusiasm either in the world of nature or in his faith in God; but he utters his pitiful laments at being cut off both from nature and from God. Nor can he make any further use of sprung rhythm; but for the most part, while he retains a deep poetic inspiration, he has to fall back on running rhythm. Thus in what seems to have been the last of his 1885 poems, "My own heart", he vainly urges himself to "not live this tormented mind/ With this tormented mind tormenting yet". The rhythm is here quite regular and running, but it is as it were running round and round in circles within the prison of his mind, as he is engaged in tormenting his already tormented mind by means of that same tormented mind. It goes on and on endlessly, as "thoughts against thoughts in groans grind" in a condition he even compares to that of the souls in hell.

Meanwhile, what about the third way I have mentioned, that of "excellence", rising above the opposition of affirmation and negation? It is what we find in Hopkins's new poem, the exceptionally long sonnet with the exceptionally long title "That Nature is a Heraclitean Fire and of the comfort of the Resurrection", which he composed after a walk on a windy day in Phoenix Park, Dublin, on July 26, 1888—less than a year before his death. Most of the sonnet is devoted to the Heraclitean idea of all things being in a state of flux, ever rising up from earth through water and air to fire, and ever falling from fire through air and water to earth again. In the world of nature, as Heraclitus taught, "the way up and the way down are one and the same". But in the world of man, in his unique individuality, it seems that "death blots black out" every mark of him, and "vastness blurs and time beats level" everything about him.

Then suddenly the poet exclaims, "Enough! The Resurrection"—not only that of Christ which took place two thousand years ago, but that in which the poet hopes to be united with Christ on the last day. Then, he says, "In a flash, at a trumpet crash"—as though recalling his phrase in stanza 8 of "The Wreck", "Brim, in a flash, full" (where "in a flash" has to be read literally in a flash, as a series of unstressed syllables between the stresses on "brim" and "full"). And he goes on, "I am all at once what Christ is, since he was what I am, and/ This Jack, joke, poor potsherd, patch, matchwood, immortal diamond,/ Is immortal diamond." That is to say, in the resurrection of the body, which will take place, as St. Paul says, at the sound of a trumpet and in the twinkling of an eye, he will find himself risen like Christ, even as Christ in his earthly life had assumed a mortal body like that of Hopkins. And then all that is inferior in him, all that makes him a mere "Jack, joke, poor potsherd, patch, matchwood", disguising the "immortal diamond" of his spirit, will fall away and reveal what St. Paul calls "a spiritual body".

Such is the vision Hopkins comes to see at the end of his earthly life and his poetic career, and to express in this culminating poem of 1888, as it were recapitulating what he had seen and expressed in the vision of the nun in "The Wreck", the vision of Christ coming to her and her sisters with compassion "in the storm of his strides". And such is the vision which was realized for him when the time came for him to die of typhus fever at the young age of 44 in June 1889. Then, in spite of his preceding complaints of being "Time's eunuch" and not being able to "breed one work that wakes", he is said to have repeated in his dying words, "I am so happy". And so he died, unknown to most of his contemporaries, without having been able to publish any of his great poems to "the yet knowing world". Only some thirty years later, his friend Robert Bridges—to whom he had sent copies of all his poems, only to receive uncomprehending criticism, yet who in the course of time came to be crowned England's poet laureate—arranged for his poems to be published in 1918 by the Oxford University Press. And so Hopkins's poetic message came to be heard, at first only by those whom Milton calls "fit audience though but few", but later, especially after World War II and the publication of the third edition of *Poems* in 1948, by men in every land even to the ends of the earth—even to this land of Japan.

(*Hopkins Research* 24, December 1995)

"The Dearest Freshness"

"Dear . . . fresh . . . sweet . . ." What sentimental, wishy-washy words they are! And how typical of the poetic vocabulary of Hopkins! Had he lived in our hard-boiled, frost-bitten age, he would soon have been warned off them, before ever he came to use them in his poems. Such words all too easily cloy, cloud, and sour, as the poet himself indirectly admits in the case of "innocent mind and Mayday in girl and boy". But in themselves and in their original meaning they are perfectly good, containing in them what the poet calls "a strain of the earth's sweet being in the beginning/ In Eden garden". It is only as a result of original sin that they come to cloy, cloud, and sour—not so much in the mind of the poet using them as in that of the critic frowning on his use of them.

There is something these three words have deeply in common in the poet's mind. They express both what he finds in the world of nature in springtime and what he finds in himself as he responds to that world. Concerning it he exclaims in "God's Grandeur", "There lives the dearest freshness deep down things"; and this is what he identifies in "Spring" as the above-mentioned "strain of the earth's sweet being in the beginning". It is what he sees, to begin with, in plants and flowers in the season of spring, particularly in the morning. It is what he sees in the vase of flowers, "Fetched fresh, as I suppose, off some sweet wood" and placed "at very entering" not only of the "house where all were good" to him but also of the poem describing that house. It is what he sees in the "fresh-firecoal chestnut-falls" among the examples of "Pied Beauty", which are subsequently echoed in the "wet-fresh windfalls of war's storm" in "To what serves Mortal Beauty?" It is what he sees in his "aspens dear" with their "fresh and following folded rank", whose felling he laments in "Binsey Poplars".

It is, above all, what he sees in human beings in their age of innocence and their Mayday of life. It is what he sees in "the sweetest air" of the little hero of "The Handsome Heart". It is what he sees in the "freshyouth fretted in a bloomfall" of the bugler boy to whom he gives his "First Communion", while anticipating "that sweet's sweeter ending". It is what he sees in the "sweet scions", to be bred "out of hallowed bodies", as he fondly anticipates in "At the Wedding March". It is what he sees not only in childhood but also in sickness, when the sick revert as it were to their second childhood and are born again, as in "Felix Randal", the one-time strong and sturdy farrier, to whom in his last sickness the priest-poet tendered "our sweet reprieve and ransom" in holy communion. Then, he reflects, "This seeing the sick endears them to us, us too it endears."

All the same, it remains true that this springtime freshness in nature and man is all too frail and flowing, like "the fleeciest, frailest-flixed snowflake", so delicate and so "rife in every least thing's life", but all too ready to melt with the rising of the sun. It is, as the poet laments in "The Golden Echo", "whatever's prized and passes of us, everything that's fresh and fast flying of us, seems to us sweet of us and swiftly away with, done away with, undone . . . yet dearly and dangerously sweet of us . . . fastened with the tenderest truth to its own best being and its loveliness of youth". It is, in other words, an object at once of the poet's fond contemplation, in which he would like to remain forever, and of his fonder lamentation, as he observes at the beginning of Part II of "The Wreck", how "Flesh falls within sight of us". Then he can't help wondering what he can do about it, apart from wringing his hands or the barriers of his cage (as he puts it in "The Caged Skylark") "in bursts of fear or rage".

This is a problem to which Hopkins recurs more than once in his poems, and in which he rises well above the imputation of mere aestheticism which he might otherwise have incurred. He recurs to it in his significantly entitled poem, "Morning, Midday, and Evening Sacrifice", as he dwells on "all this beauty blooming" and "all this freshness fuming", before coming to the conclusion, "Give God while worth consuming." He recurs to it at greater length in "The Golden Echo", where, after dwelling on the frailty and transience of mortal beauty, he insists on the importance of sacrifice, that is, of giving "beauty back, beauty, beauty, beauty, back to God", as being "beauty's self and beauty's giver", by whom "the thing we freely forfeit is kept with fonder a care, fonder a care kept than we could have kept it".

Here precisely is the point at which the poetry of Hopkins leads to the deep theological vision of what he calls in one of his spiritual writings "The Great Sacrifice". The ideal of sacrifice, which he requires of himself and his readers in response to mortal beauty, is what he shows from the beginning in the eternal procession of the Son from the Father. "Why," he asks, "did the Son of God go forth from the Father not only in the eternal and intrinsic procession of the Trinity but also by an extrinsic and less than eternal, let us say aeonian one?" And he answers, "To give God glory and that by sacrifice, sacrifice offered in the barren wilderness outside of God, as the children of Israel were led into the wilderness to offer sacrifice." And he continues, "This sacrifice and this outward procession is a consequence and shadow of the procession of the Trinity, from which mystery sacrifice takes its rise. . . . It is as if the blissful agony or stress of selving in God had forced out drops of sweat or blood."

This is all very mysterious; but it is a mystery that helps to explain the other, poetic mystery in Part I of "The Wreck". Here the poet speaks of a mysterious "bliss" and "stress": the bliss, which he feels as he gazes up at a "starlight night" and even kisses his hand "To the stars, lovely-asunder starlight", he sees wafting the divine presence "out of it"; and the stress, which is somehow "under the world's splendour and wonder". He also speaks of a "stroke and a stress that stars and storms deliver", leading "the faithful" to waver, and "the faithless" to fable and miss. In his theological vision, as here expressed in poetic form, "It dates from day/ Of his going in Galilee", that is to say, from the moment of his incarnation, subsequently described in the same poem as "the heaven-flung, heart-fleshed, maiden-furled/ Miracle-in-Mary-of-flame". Such is the way Hopkins rephrases the *Verbum Supernum Prodiens* of St. Thomas Aquinas—the supernal Word proceeding without departing from the Father's right hand. From this first moment of the incarnation he himself proceeds almost at once to the final moment of the redemption and sacrifice in "The dense and the driven Passion, and frightful sweat".

But that isn't all. What he sees in his poetic and theological vision, in the world not only of nature and man but even of God, Hopkins has to experience for himself in the subsequent agony of his priestly and poetic life. His earlier prayer for "thy creature dear" in "In the Valley of the Elwy" and for "dear and dogged man" in the other valley of "Ribblesdale" is answered only too painfully in his own case as he turns to pray for "Patience": "We hear our hearts grate on themselves: it kills/ To bruise them dearer. Yet the rebellious wills/ Of us we do bid God bend to him even so." Now it is his turn to lie like Felix Randal on a more than metaphorical bed of sickness, in which the poems it evokes sound almost like curses. Now from "sweet" he feels only the taste of "bitter", even to the extent of adding, "My taste was me", while recalling how "Bones built in me, flesh filled, blood brimmed the curse." Now the "Selfyeast of spirit" in him, once so fresh and dear to him, is but a source of sourness to the "dull dough" of his flesh. Now it is as if what has been "bonniest, dearest" to nature in himself is quenched and "all is in an enormous dark/ Drowned".

Yet it is precisely in such a moment of "dark descending", amid lightning and winter, that God most reveals himself as "Father and fondler of heart thou hast wrung" and is most merciful—both as Father to son and as Creator to creature. Then what the poet has already recognized, if theoretically, in the two parts of "The Wreck", he goes on to experience all of a sudden in his own case in his longest sonnet, with its proportionally long title, "That Nature is a Heraclitean Fire and of the comfort of the Resurrection". Here the "enormous dark" of death, emphasized by the rhyme-words "mark" and "stark", is immediately countered with the resolute "Enough! The Resurrection." Here, too, the poet isn't content with merely looking to the vision, now no longer merely poetic or theological but personal, of the risen Christ. He explicitly looks back to his earlier poem as he compares his situation to that of a "foundering deck" across which there now shines "a beacon, an eternal beam". Such is the vision of Christ experienced by the nun in "The Wreck": "There then! the Master,/ *Ipse*, the only one, Christ, King, Head", who appears to her as "a blown beacon of light" and as "Jesu, heart's light".

Now the poet feels he may well let "Flesh fade, and mortal trash/ Fall to the residuary worm". For all is but mortal beauty, destined to fall "within sight of us". It is for him to "leave, let that alone", as he advises in the end of his sonnet "To what serves Mortal Beauty?" All is what he has already freely given up and offered in sacrifice at morning, midday, and evening. But now all that was merely mortal he retrieves on a higher, purer, nobler level, transformed into "God's better beauty, grace", as in his own resurrection he finds himself "all at once what Christ is, since he was what I am", namely, "immortal diamond".

Such, in short, is "the dearest freshness" that Hopkins finds "deep down things", in the grandeur of God shining down through the incarnate Word of Christ over the "bright wings" of the Holy Ghost. Even more shortly, it is what he expresses in the climax of his sonnet "God's Grandeur" with the exclamation of enlightenment, "Ah!"

(*Hopkins Research* 25, December 1996)

Hamlet *in Hopkins*

By the magic of his words, Shakespeare, like his own Prospero, exercises a strange fascination over the minds and words of Englishmen from generation to generation. It is almost impossible for anyone who has been exposed to that influence from childhood to escape from it in later life. The plays of Shakespeare, as they drew upon almost every form of influence in his own time, continue to exercise their own influence in after-time. Poets such as Hopkins and Eliot even complain of this influence, the former even going so far as to say in one of his letters that the example of Shakespeare "has done ever so much harm by his very genius". But the harm is far outweighed by the good, as Hopkins's own example may serve to reassure us. In all his poems Hopkins can hardly forbear betraying what he calls the "underthought" of Shakespeare, especially from the four great tragedies, including *Hamlet*. So now, concentrating on this one play, let me examine how deeply its underthought has entered into Hopkins's mature poems from "The Wreck" onwards, and how in consequence the poet may be seen in these poems as a commentator on the play, from act to act and from scene to scene.

ACT I: From the opening words of the play, Bernardo's expression of alarm, "Who's there?", we may note an echo in "The Lantern Out of Doors", where the poet sees a lantern moving along in the night and imagines himself challenging the bearer: "And who goes there?" The reason for Bernardo's alarm soon becomes apparent as "this thing", to wit, the ghost of the former king, when the friends suddenly break off their discussion of its appearance with Marcellus's cry, "Look, where it comes again!" This apparition is recalled in the climactic stanza 28 of "The Wreck", where the poet excitedly points across the turbulent waves from the viewpoint of the drowning nun, "Strike you the sight of it? Look at it loom there,/ Thing that she," and then he breaks off, as the phantom he sees turns out to be none other than the risen Christ.

In the ensuing discussion Horatio endeavours to give a rational explanation of the phenomenon by recalling the classic example of Caesar's death "in the most high and palmy state of Rome". Hopkins takes him up on this unusual use of "palmy" in his poem on "Henry Purcell", with the impressive image of a "great stormfowl" and his "palmy snow-pinions"—though his echo of Shakespeare's metaphorical use of this epithet is more literal, serving to "fan fresh our wits with wonder".

Turning to the second scene, we may notice how many of Hopkins's poems recall passages from Hamlet's opening soliloquy, "O that this too too solid flesh would melt!" The prince's lament over "the uses of this world", as "weary, stale, flat and unprofitable", is aptly echoed in the poet's Dublin sonnet, "To seem the stranger", where he describes himself as "weary of idle a being". And his concluding words, "But break, my heart, for I must hold my tongue!", are further echoed by the poet in a letter to his mother about this time: "The grief of mind that I go through over politics, over what I read and hear and see in Ireland about England, is such that I can neither express it nor bear to speak of it." Where Hamlet recalls how his mother would "hang on" his father, Hopkins reverses the genders in his sonnet on the afflicted Church, "Andromeda", imagining how Christ as Perseus "hangs his thoughts on her". Then in contrast Hamlet laments how his mother has changed now that his father is "but two months dead, nay, not so much, not two"; while in Hopkins's "Binsey Poplars" there is a similar self-correction forced out of the poet's deep feelings, "Not spared, not one." Hamlet's subsequent outcry, "Why she, even she", is also paralleled in "Binsey Poplars", in the poet's complaint, "Where we, even where we mean/ To mend her, we end her."

Later on in the same scene, when Horatio comes to inform the young Hamlet of his father's apparition, he speaks of the time as "the dead vast and middle of the night"; and we find this recalled by Hopkins in "Spelt from Sibyl's Leaves", in his solemn description of night as "time's vast", where commentators are divided over the interpretation of "vast", whether as a noun (as Shakespeare here uses it) or an adjective. As for the climax of the act, when the ghost actually appears and speaks to Hamlet, we may find not a few echoes in Hopkins's poems. Thus where the ghost refers to "the secrets of my prison-house", the poet speaks of spirits "pent in prison" in stanza 33 of "The Wreck". And where the ghost further laments how he was "cut off even in the blossoms of my sin,/ Unhousel'd, disappointed, unanel'd" and so "Sent to my account/ with all my imperfections on my head", the poet laments in "The Loss of the Eurydice" how many of the sailors were "asleep unawakened, all un-/ warned" of the disaster, just as in "The Wreck" he speaks with regret of "the comfortless unconfessed of them".

∽

ACT II: In Act II, however, the only word of Hamlet I find echoed by Hopkins is that in which he confesses his despondency about man: "And yet, to me, what is this quintessence of dust? Man delights not me." Something of this feeling comes out in stanza 11 of "The Wreck", where the poet indignantly exclaims of man's obtuseness about his human condition, "But we dream we are rooted in earth—Dust!" Again, in his further expression of disgust in "The shepherd's brow", the poet cries, "But man—we scaffold of score brittle bones", and "Man Jack the man is, just"—where "just" includes an implicit rhyme with "dust". (One might also point to a further echo of Isabella's words to Angelo in *Measure for Measure*, "But man, proud man. . . .")

∽

ACT III: Almost inevitably, when we come to Hamlet's great soliloquy of "To be, or not to be", we find several echoes in the poems of Hopkins. The opening question is recalled by him in "Carrion Comfort", as he chooses the former alternative, at least by not choosing the latter, "not choose not to be"—which is what Hamlet, too, effectively chooses. As for Hamlet's equation of "to die" with "to sleep", as offering some comfort, this recurs in the dark sonnet "No worst" (which interestingly follows the underthought of *King Lear*), in the final line, "All life death does end and each day dies with sleep." Then the "heartache" of Hamlet seems to be echoed in "the sodden-with-its-sorrowing heart" in stanza 27 of "The Wreck". And Hamlet's "mortal coil" is recalled in "all that coil" of "Carrion Comfort". Again, the second mention by Hamlet of "a weary life" points to Hopkins "weary of idle a being" in "To seem the stranger". Then, after the painful dialogue between Hamlet and Ophelia in what is called "the nunnery scene", when Hamlet is recalled by the poor heroine as "the expectancy and rose of the fair state", this unusual epithet is applied by Hopkins to Christ in the concluding stanza of "The Wreck": "Pride, rose, prince, hero of us."

Jumping now over the scene of the play-within-the-play, we come to the great scene with the soliloquy of Claudius's would-be repentance. Here "the primal eldest curse" mentioned by Claudius, the curse of Cain, is recalled by Hopkins in stanza 20 of "The Wreck", where he notes: "From life's dawn it is drawn down,/ Abel is Cain's brother and breasts they have sucked the same." Where the king goes on to complain, "Pray can I not", he is numbering himself among "the past-prayer" though not yet "penitent" spirits mentioned in stanza 33. And where he goes on to refer to God as "above", he may be echoed in stanza 21, "But thou art above." There, Claudius adds, "the action lies in his true nature", which is what Hopkins also recognizes in "Spelt from Sibyl's Leaves", in the stark contrast between "black, white; right, wrong", when one is "ware of a world where but these two tell".

There follows the other great closet scene between Hamlet and his mother, in which Hamlet's memory of his father, "Where every god did seem to set his seal", may be traced in Hopkins's "O-seal-that-so feature"—which may also be seen as a distant echo of Florizel's delighted description of Perdita in *The Winter's Tale*, "What you do/ Still betters what is done." Then, more clearly, his mention of "rank corruption, mining all within" is echoed in stanza 4 of "The Wreck", in "Mined with a motion".

∽

ACT IV: Here, as in Act II, there is a decline of dramatic intensity and of memorable scenes, as also of Hopkinsian echoes. Only one occurs to my mind, in the queen's description of Hamlet's dangerous behaviour, "Mad as the sea and wind, when both contend/ Which is the mightier"—where Hopkins speaks in "Felix Randal" of "Fatal four disorders" as "fleshed there" and "all contending" for the sick man.

∽

ACT V: So we come to the final act and the end of the final scene, when in his dying moments Hamlet requests his friend Horatio, "In this harsh world draw thy breath in pain/ To tell my story." Such is the condition of man as portrayed by Hopkins in "The shepherd's brow", where he morbidly anticipates "hoary/ Age gasp; whose breath is our *memento mori*". Then, as soon as Hamlet has breathed his last gasp, in comes Fortinbras with the astonished exclamation, "This quarry cries on havoc. O proud Death,/ What feast is toward in thine eternal cell?" Such is Hopkins's lament in "Binsey Poplars" on how "Strokes of havoc unselve/ The sweet especial scene"; and such is his cry in "Carrion Comfort": "Not, I'll not, carrion comfort, Despair, not feast on thee." Thus he seems to be drawing an implicit contrast between Hamlet's half-hearted "To be, or not to be", which only leads to this feast of Death, and his own resolution "not choose not to be" and not to admit of any feast of Despair.

In the foregoing comments I have but drawn attention to various places in Hopkins's poems where he seems to be influenced by memories of Shakespeare's *Hamlet*. More precisely, I have gone through that play in detail, showing how often the poet seems to be recalling Shakespearean phrases. As for the conclusion to be drawn from it all, all I can say for the present is that Hopkins seems to have made his own much of Hamlet's character as well as his language. But in the outcome, as Hopkins found himself engulfed by a problem strangely similar to that of Shakespeare's young prince (as also of the old king in *King Lear*) he convulsively shook off the melancholy of Hamlet (as also the despair of Lear) with an affirmation not only of being, in "Carrion Comfort", but also of faith, in "That Nature is a Heraclitean Fire, and of the comfort of the Resurrection".

(*Hopkins Research* 26, December 1997)

Twin Beacons in the Life of Hopkins

It was no accident that prompted Hopkins to break his seven years of poetic silence during his theological studies at St. Beuno's College in North Wales. In one sense, of course, it *was* an accident, namely the sad shipwreck of the *Deutschland* at the mouth of the Thames in the icy waters of the North Sea. Yet in his poetic portrayal of that shipwreck, the poet looks back to something deep in his own life evoked by the seeming accident, a moment of "now done darkness" when "in lightning and lashed rod" he confessed to feeling the mysterious finger of divine providence.

Now what, we may ask, was this moment in the poet's life? Was it perhaps the moment of his conversion, when in his undergraduate days at Oxford he decided to move from "The Half-way House" of his former Anglican Church to a new home in the Roman Catholic Church? Or was it perhaps the moment of the storm that broke with memorable intensity as well over the college of St. Beuno's—as we find recorded in the beadle's log-book—as over the *Deutschland* at the mouth of the Thames? Or may we not say, with T. S. Eliot, that it was rather "a lifetime burning in every moment", a string of such moments of storm and stress followed by calm, such as Hopkins implies in one of his darkest sonnets, "But where I say/ Hours, I mean years, mean life"?

In each of these moments, whether one or many, or a succession of many seen as one, we may say that out of the poet's darkness there shines a heavenly light—just as when in the first day of creation God said, "Let there be light", and there was light. This is what the poet represents the nun in "The Wreck" as experiencing amid "Wind's burly and beat of endragoned seas", when she sees and in turn becomes "a blown beacon of light". This is also what he subsequently sees and becomes when, at the end of his dark Dublin period, he declares in the very jaws of despair, "Across my foundering deck shone/ A beacon, an eternal beam."

Now what, we may further ask, is this beacon whose shining characterizes the poet's successive moments of shipwreck and salvation—or, to use the terms of Newman's alternative, of loss and gain? In one sense, this question may seem a needless one; since in the context of the two poems in which the "beacon" appears, it is clearly the divine light that first shone over the waters of chaos in the first day of creation. It is the light mentioned by John Henry Newman in the opening line of his hymn, "Lead, kindly light, amid the encircling gloom"—the hymn that Hopkins himself wrote out in full in his diary for 1865. But it is also the light in which Newman himself was sharing with his characteristic idea of "two luminous beings", God and himself. So for Hopkins, too, it may be said that Newman was also for him such a beacon of light.

Then how did Newman become a beacon of light for Hopkins? There was, of course, to begin with, the abovementioned hymn, which is entitled "The Pillar of Cloud", and which Hopkins also echoes in his poem "Nondum" in Lent 1866. We may further note how in the title of his other poem of this time, "The Half-way House", dated October 1865, he echoes Newman's statement in the *Apologia pro Vita Sua*, which he had evidently been reading, that the Anglican Church was but a half-way house on the road to Rome. This was, we may well conclude, the light that was guiding the steps of Hopkins, when he first approached Newman in his sudden letter of August 28, 1866, expressing his longing "to become a Catholic", then visited Newman at the Birmingham Oratory in September, and finally made his formal submission to the Catholic Church at the same Oratory in Newman's presence on October 21.

This crucial moment of conversion was clearly, under God, inspired by the "kindly light" of Newman, as manifested not only in the hymn and the *Apologia*, but also and above all in his person, as described by Hopkins to his friend Bridges at this time, "most kind . . . genial and almost, so to speak, unserious . . . so sensible". From then onwards Newman may be regarded as the spiritual father, if not angel guardian, of Hopkins, who in his letters to Newman regularly signed himself, "Your affectionate son in Christ".

But now, we may ask, what was the further influence of Newman, as a "beacon of light", not only on the life but also on the poetry of Hopkins? There is no doubt that Newman guided him in his decision to seek admission into the Society of Jesus, in spite or because of its "hard discipline", though not in his other decision to sacrifice his existing poems and even his hopes of further poetic composition. Still, once Hopkins had entered the Society, he came under other guidance than Newman's; and so in his letters to Newman we find his relations with his former guide becoming more distant, not to say cool. In poetry, too, however much he may have admired Newman's "Lead, kindly light", he subsequently came to dismiss his poetic achievement, in a letter to Canon Dixon, as marking the expiry of the Lake School of poets, together with Keble and Faber. In prose, while praising Newman as "our greatest master of style" in a letter to Edward Bond, he later criticized him, in a letter to Coventry Patmore, for shirking "the technic of written prose" and for shunning "the tradition of written English".

All the same, in the above-mentioned letter to Edward Bond, Hopkins does speak with enthusiasm of Newman's *Grammar of Assent*, commending in particular "the justice and candour and gravity and rightness of mind . . . in all he writes"—though he admits "it is perhaps heavy reading". He even went on to suggest in his birthday letter to Newman for 1883 that he be allowed to write a commentary on the book. What he might have written is an interesting matter for speculation; but unfortunately Newman seems to have taken his proposal as implying a criticism of its obscurity, and so he turned it down as unnecessary. Evidently, Hopkins was tactless, and Newman was oversensitive.

No less speculative is the matter of Newman's influence on Hopkins's mature poetry from "The Wreck" onwards. In his biography *Gerard Manley Hopkins*, Bernard Bergonzi notes "the significant moment" when on September 20, 1866, Hopkins met Newman, calling it "the first meeting of the two greatest Catholic writers in English of the nineteenth century". But alas, the "beacon of light" which Hopkins had seen in Newman from a distance came to be diminished on closer personal acquaintance and on the subsequent divergence of their paths—though the former eventually followed the latter's footsteps to what he recognized, in a letter to Newman himself, as "a university for Catholic Ireland begun under your leadership". At least, we may add, what Hopkins was now to experience for himself in Dublin was, in his earlier words to another Oxford friend, Edward Urquhart, in 1868, "the silence and the severity of God, as Dr. Newman very eloquently and persuasively has said in a passage of the Anglican Difficulties".

Here we may turn back to Hopkins's diary for 1865, for yet another "beacon of light", in the form of a transcription of a prose passage from J. C. Shairp's essay on Wordsworth's "spots of time", which had appeared the previous year in the *North British Review*. The passage reads as follows:

> Each scene in nature has in it a power of awakening, in every beholder of sensibility, an impression peculiar to itself, such as no other scene can exactly call up. This may be called the "heart" or "character" of that scene. It is quite analogous to, if somewhat vaguer than, the particular impression produced upon us by the presence of each individual man. Now the aggregate of the impressions produced by many scenes in nature, or rather the power in nature on a large scale of producing such impressions, is what, for want of another name, I have called the "heart" of nature.

Here we may recognize, in more general terms, what Hopkins more specially and even technically came to call "inscape", for the particular impression, and "instress", for the power in nature of producing such impressions. Even at this time he was writing his fragmentary essay on Parmenides, in which he makes use of these favourite terms of his for the first time—"inscape" four times, "instress" three times, and "stress" twice. It is surely a remarkable coincidence!

As for the "spots of time", which Wordsworth mentions in his *Prelude* as "moments . . . scattered everywhere", endowed with a "renovating virtue", we may note the special influence of the earlier poet on the later, not least in his ode on "Intimations of Immortality". On many if not most of his other poems Hopkins is particularly harsh in his judgment, because, as he tells his friend Baillie, "he writes such an intolerable deal of Parnassian"—by which he means "the language of poetry draping prose thought". But on this one poem of Wordsworth's Hopkins has nothing but praise, particularly in a letter to Canon Dixon, defending it against his friend's criticism. In certain great men, he remarks, at certain times, "human nature . . . saw something, got a shock, wavers in opinion, looking back, whether there was anything in it or no, but is in a tremble ever since." Now, he adds, "in Wordsworth, when he wrote that ode, human nature got another of those shocks, and the tremble from it is spreading. This opinion I do strongly share; I am, ever since I knew the ode, in a tremble." Moreover, he commends the ode as "better than anything else I know of Wordsworth", considering that "the interest and importance of the matter was here of the highest, his insight was at its very deepest".

Here, in the case of Wordsworth, as contrasted with that of Newman—for all the latter's ideal of heart speaking to heart—we have poet speaking to poet. However great Newman's spiritual influence may have been on Hopkins in his religious conversion, when it comes to matters of poetry and "spiritual insight into nature", Wordsworth's influence, as "a blown beacon of light", seems to be the greater on Hopkins's mature poetry from "The Wreck" onwards.

In particular, we may note two phrases from Wordsworth's ode that evidently so impressed Hopkins that he commented on them in his above-mentioned letter to Dixon. The magical change he notes in "O joy that in our embers" may be echoed in stanza 23 of "The Wreck", beginning "Joy fall to thee, father Francis", and ending with "his all-fire glances"—the joy, I mean, that comes out of the all-consuming fire of divine love. This joy is not only everywhere apparent in this poem of shipwreck, which is applied as much to the poet himself as to the five nuns, but it also spills over into his characteristic sonnet "The Windhover", in which he echoes both this stanza of "The Wreck" and the "embers" of Wordsworth's ode. Indeed, in the climax of his sonnet, he leads up to the mention of "bluebleak embers" as they "fall, gall themselves, and gash goldvermilion". It is almost as if the poet has written the sonnet in unconscious tribute to the earlier ode.

The other phrase on which Hopkins comments is what he calls Wordsworth's stroke, "steeped in beauty and yearning", namely, "The moon doth with delight". Here we may recall his lesser known poem entitled "Moonrise", dated June 19, 1876, in which the poet describes the moon as "lovely in waning but lustreless", rising above "dark Maenefa the mountain" behind St. Beuno's College. "This," he exclaims, "was the prized, the desirable sight, unsought, presented so easily"—as it were one of Wordsworth's "spots of time". In the same passage, Wordsworth goes on to speak of "a starry night", which, more than the sight of the moon, evokes the wonder of the later poet. Thus in stanza 5 of "The Wreck" Hopkins expresses his joy in "the world's splendour and wonder", or rather in the divine mystery within it, in terms of "the stars, lovely-asunder/ Starlight, wafting him out of it". And in his subsequent sonnet on "The Starlight Night" he exclaims with the enthusiastic delight of a child, "Look at the stars! look, look up at the skies!"

One might well go through all Hopkins's poems from "The Wreck" onwards, seeking in them varied echoes of Wordsworth's "Immortality Ode". One might, for instance, begin from the beginning, from the opening line, "There was a time when meadow, grove, and stream", and point to the similar-sounding enumeration in "In the Valley of the Elwy": "Lovely the woods, waters, meadows, combes, vales." Wordsworth here makes no mention of "waters", but later on in his ode he speaks of "the mighty waters". Hopkins, too, goes on to speak of man in this setting as "the inmate", as if following the hint from Wordsworth, who also speaks of "her inmate, Man". Moreover, Wordsworth's emphasis from the outset of his ode is on "the glory and the freshness of a dream", as he once saw the earth around him in his childhood. So Hopkins looks in stanza 5 of "The Wreck" to "the world's splendour and wonder", where he also echoes the other words of the ode, "Of splendour in the grass, of glory in the flower". Then in the subsequent sonnet on "God's Grandeur", he admires how "The world is charged with the grandeur of God", adding that, in spite of everything man can do to the contrary, "There lives the dearest freshness deep down things". Even "the clouds that gather round the setting sun" in Wordsworth's ode seem to be recalled in "the last lights" that "off the black west went"; and it may be added that the "immortality" that "broods like the day" over Wordsworth's child looks forward to "the Holy Ghost" who "over the bent world broods with warm breast and with ah! bright wings".

One might say that Wordsworth's ode as a whole, with its abrupt contrasts between darkness and light, death and life, time and eternity, is developed, through occasional possible/probable echoes, in the whole corpus of Hopkins's mature poetry. For example, we may note "the racing lambs" in "Spring", the "grieving" of Margaret in "Spring and Fall", the "cataracts" in "Inversnaid", the month of May in "The May Magnificat", the "innocent mind and Mayday in girl and boy" in "Spring", the "faith that looks through death" in

"That Nature is a Heraclitean Fire", with its triumphant vindication of "the Resurrection". Even Wordsworth's concluding emphasis on "the human heart by which we live", with its "thoughts that do often lie too deep for tears", seems to be taken up by Hopkins at a crucial turning point of "The Wreck", as he pauses to reflect on the "mother of being in me, heart", which surprises him with "tears, is it? Tears".

Comparing the two poets with each other, however, we have to admit that what is vague and general in Wordsworth becomes precise and particular in Hopkins; what is merely philosophical and even pantheistic in Wordsworth becomes more clearly theological and Christian in Hopkins; what is seen as "divine" and "spiritual" in Wordsworth becomes more definitely related to the three persons in God, Father, Son, and Spirit, in Hopkins; behind Wordsworth's "Nature" Hopkins sees the mantle of "the mighty mother", Mary. Still, the latter poet pays a handsome tribute to his predecessor when he goes on in his letter to Dixon to affirm: "I think St. George and St. Thomas of Canterbury wore roses in heaven for England's sake on the day that ode, not without their intercession, was penned."

In conclusion, it may seem as if the influence of Wordsworth on Hopkins's poetry has to be considered as greater than that of Newman. Or rather, it may seem as if what had begun in the mind of Hopkins when he transcribed Newman's hymn "Lead, kindly light" was brought to completion in his mature poetry by his admiration for Wordsworth's "Immortality" ode. If we may say that their respective influences were twin "beacons of light" in his life, must we not also say that the beacon of Wordsworth is brighter than that of Newman? Such a comparison may well seem odious; but the odium may, I submit, be removed by a simple distinction. It is, after all, only natural that the poetry of Wordsworth, in particular his "Immortality" ode, should have exercised a more conscious influence on the mature poetry of Hopkins. But that isn't the same as saying that Wordsworth exercised a deeper influence on Hopkins's life. That remained the prerogative of Newman, even after Hopkins's entrance into the Society of Jesus, not least when the poet came to experience for himself "the silence and the severity of God" during his Dublin years, not long after he had made his proposal to write a commentary on Newman's *Grammar of Assent*. For when we reflect on the implicit point of the *Grammar*, we may see it as arising out of the author's own assent to the Church of Rome, and thereby influencing Hopkins's subsequent assent, as the heart of one spoke to the heart of the other. And in either case, we may add, it was an assent not made just once but renewed from moment to moment as what T. S. Eliot calls "a lifetime burning in every moment".

(*Hopkins Research* 27, December 1998)

Hopkins and the Imagery of Procreation

It may seem strange for a poet like Hopkins, who wasn't merely a bachelor but a Jesuit poet bound by the vow of chastity, to have made the imagery of procreation so central to his poetic oeuvre, so central indeed that there is hardly another poet in the English language to compare with him in this respect save perhaps his poetic friend and correspondent Coventry Patmore. Yet so it is. And the poem of his in which this imagery stands out most vividly isn't anything he wrote before his entry into religious life in 1868, but that with which he broke his "elected silence" some seven years later in poetic commemoration of a shipwreck at the mouth of the Thames in 1875.

What, we may wonder, is the connection between shipwreck and procreation? The two images seem to be as far apart from each other as death is from life. Yet for Hopkins it was precisely out of this incident of shipwreck and the accompanying loss of life—"of a fourth the doom to be drowned"—that he felt a new poetic inspiration coming down upon him as if from heaven, even from the "finger of God's right hand"—as the Holy Spirit is invoked in the hymn, *Veni Creator Spiritus*: "Over again I feel thy finger and find thee."

Then what, we may further ask, was so inspiring to Hopkins in the loss of so many lives on board the ill-fated *Deutschland*? At that time the poet might well have read accounts of the loss of many other lives in other shipwrecks around the rocky coastline of England. What, then, was so "counter, original, spare, strange" about this one? It was because among the two hundred passengers and crew on board there were five Franciscan nuns going into exile from their convent home in Germany to a new world in America, and they were all five of them drowned. For them the poet felt a deep surge of fraternal sympathy, as he exclaims concerning one of them, their leader: "Sister, a sister calling/ A master, her master and mine." What is more, it was this call of "the tall nun" that most profoundly affected him in the newspaper accounts of the wreck and led him to compose his poem. Not that he was drawn to her by any sex appeal, as Freudian critics might imagine, but that he saw her as drawn to Christ, her and his divine spouse. The climax of his description of her comes in stanza 28, where in a series of excited, broken sentences he imagines Christ coming to her over the waters and taking her to himself, as in a mystic marriage of bridegroom and bride whose imagery is at the heart of the poem.

This imagery is made explicit in the following stanza 29, in which the ecstasy of union between bridegroom and bride leads to the moment of conception: "For so conceived, so to conceive thee is done." This is an immaculate conception not of the body but of the mind, as the sister with "heart right" and "single eye" is enabled to read "the unshapeable shock night" and to know "the who and the why". This imagery leads the poet to reflect further on the occasion of the shipwreck and this union of the nun with her divine spouse. For providentially, as he notes, the feast that "followed the night thou hadst glory of this nun" was none other than that of the Immaculate Conception, the "feast of the one woman without stain", on December 8. Here Mary is seen not only as mother of Jesus, to whom she gave virgin birth following on the message of the angel, but also as spouse of the Word from the beginning, even from the moment of her own conception, the Word she heard and kept and uttered outright in the fullness of time.

All this isn't just seen and represented objectively by the poet in the second part of his poem, but he also applies it subjectively to himself in the first part, which he may have composed—as Sir Thomas More is said to have composed his *Utopia*—after the second part, by way of personal preface. In it he looks back to a similar if metaphorical moment of shipwreck and mystical union in his own life, which may have been the moment of his religious conversion to the Church of Rome. When that moment came, as he told a friend, it came all of a sudden, yet, as he says in stanza 34, "not a doomsday dazzle in his coming nor dark as he came", but "kind" and "royally reclaiming his own".

All the same, the way the poet describes this experience in the first part does look like a dark doomsday, as he recalls how "I did say yes/ O at lightning and lashed rod". He feels the terror of Christ descending on him with "the sweep and the hurl" of some monstrous creature that "trod hard down with a horror of height". It recalls the mythological terror of Leda subsequently portrayed by W. B. Yeats in terms of the "sudden blow" from the wings of the divine Swan, as the poor girl endures a combined rape and rapture, "mastered by the brute blood of the air", or of the "threefold terror of love" imagined by the same poet in the case of "The Mother of God", as she bears "the terror of all terrors" in her womb. In Hopkins's poem, however, there is no unwilling response to the irruption of the divine but a willing assent, as in the wedding ceremony: "I did say yes." Thereupon the seeming storm is succeeded by a miraculous calm, as the poet goes on to say of himself, "I am soft sift . . . steady as a water in a well, to a poise, to a pane," and to "kiss my hand/ To the stars, lovely-asunder/ Starlight, wafting him out of it."

Such, too, he sees, is the moment "of his going in Galilee", when the virginal conception of Jesus by Mary through her willing response to the angelic annunciation leads successively to the "warm-laid grave of a womb-life grey", the birth in a "manger", and the child laid on the "maiden's knee". This succession of events in the infant life of Jesus is replaced at the end of his mortal life with "The dense and the driven Passion, and frightful sweat", symbolized by the age-old storm with its providential purpose to force the human heart, "hard at bay" like a deer pursued by hounds of heaven, to come "out with it" and to "lash with the best or worst/ Word last". Then it is that the poet hails the divine Father as having "thy dark descending and most art merciful then".

Such is the basic theme and recurrent imagery of procreation that runs throughout "The Wreck", but it is an imagery that, strangely enough, we find reduced in the subsequent poems, in which Hopkins's poetic inspiration is somehow "cabined, cribbed, confined" within the restricted sonnet form. True, we come upon the "ecstasy" of "The Windhover", as the bird with its "hurl and gliding" rebuffs "the big wind", and the poet in turn feels his own "heart in hiding" stirred at "the achieve of, the mastery of the thing". In his own case, however, there is only the "sheer plod" of his theological studies and their "blue-bleak embers", which, as they fall, "gall themselves" and thus (he trusts) "gash gold-vermilion"—even as the nuns in their deaths by drowning, as in a second baptism, come "to bathe in his fall-gold mercies" and "to breathe in his all-fire glances".

There is a similar moment of ecstasy in "Hurrahing in Harvest", as the poet sees in the skies of autumn the "rapturous love's greeting" of his saviour, and in "the azurous hung hills" a sign of "his world-wielding shoulder". Then in their mystical union the poet feels as if his heart "rears wings bold and bolder/ And hurls for him, O half hurls earth for him off under his feet"—looking back to the moment described in stanza 3 of "The Wreck" when he "fled with a fling of the heart to the heart of the Host".

Moreover, the outcome of such moments of ecstasy is represented by the poet in terms of a mother or father bird fostering their young in their nest. This is the image we find in "The Wreck", both in stanza 12, with the sad exclamation, "O Father, not under thy feathers", with reference to the majority of the shipwrecked victims, and in stanza 31, with the hope that these same victims, though dying "comfortless unconfessed", may yet be saved by "lovely-felicitous Providence" with the divine "finger of a tender of, O of a feathery delicacy". Then in the sonnet "God's Grandeur" there is the culminating vision of "the Holy Ghost" who "over the bent/ World broods with warm breast and with ah! bright wings". In "Spring" we are shown "Thrush's eggs" that look like "little low heavens" in the nest. Similarly, in "The May Magnificat" we are shown the "Star-eyed strawberry-breasted/ Throstle above her nested/ Cluster of bugle blue eggs thin", as she "Forms and warms the life within". So the poet proceeds from description to description of "that world of good/ Nature's motherhood", till he reaches the climax of "This ecstasy all through mothering earth", which each year reminds Mary of her "mirth till Christ's birth" and her "exultation/ In God who was her salvation."

Thus in all his bright poems from "The Wreck" onwards Hopkins makes use of the rich imagery of procreation, beginning with the ecstasy preceding the moment of conception, continuing with the calmer delight of gestation, and culminating in the joy of birth—as he declares in stanza 34 of "The Wreck": "Now burn, new born to the world." But in his later, darker poems he feels himself prevented from availing himself of it by reason of "dark heaven's baffling ban" (in "To seem the stranger"). Then he finds himself obliged to hoard his poetic word "unheard", or if heard, it remains "unheeded", and the poet is left "a lonely began". All he can do is to strain as "Time's eunuch" and "not breed one work that wakes" (in "Thou art indeed just"). In other words, the poems he writes, however inspired they may be in conception and gestation, have no outlet in printed form, even in the publications of his own Society of Jesus. And when he sends them for approval to friends such as Robert Bridges, instead of appreciation or admiration he encounters only their harsh uncomprehending criticism.

This frustration of his, Hopkins sums up in his last poem, "To R. B.", in which he presents at once a full expression of his imagery of procreation and a paradoxical lament over his lack of inspiration. First, he looks up to "the fine delight that fathers thought" which comes down from above, just as, according to St. James, "every good and perfect gift comes down from above, from the Father of lights"; and it is this, he says, that leaves the mind "a mother of immortal song". Here is also an echo of the classical imagery, with which Hopkins was long familiar, of the cosmic marriage between the sky-father Zeus or Jupiter and the earth-mother Cybele or Diana. Then the poet turns to the period of gestation, as the mind "Within her wears, bears, cares and combs" her song, as "The widow of an insight lost"—though not wholly lost. Such "sweet fire", which he identifies as "the one rapture of an inspiration", the poet longs to recapture, like "the wise thrush" in Browning's poem, but now he feels it is beyond him and he can only lament, even while finding a paradoxical inspiration in that lamentation. His is now a "winter world", but, like Shelley in his "Ode to the West Wind", he looks through that winter to a second spring, if not in this life, at least in "the comfort of the Resurrection". And so Hopkins concludes his last great poem of inspiration, "That Nature is a Heraclitean Fire", by recalling his moment of shipwreck, when across his "foundering deck shone/ A beacon, an eternal beam", the vision, "In a flash, at a trumpet crash", of his final mystical reunion with Christ.

(*Hopkins Research* 28, December 1999)

Hopkins's Commentary on Newman's Grammar

IN HIS BIRTHDAY letter of February 1883 to his spiritual father, Cardinal Newman, Hopkins proposed his hope of writing a commentary on the other's *Grammar of Assent*, which had been published many years before in 1870. Needless to say, Newman turned down the proposal, in something of a huff at the suggestion that his book was in need of a commentary. Unfortunately, what he failed to realize, owing to his excessive touchiness, was that Hopkins might have had other ideas of his own to contribute to the subject—intimately affecting as it did the life and thought of both men, central as they both were to "the second spring" of English Catholicism. What a pity, we may reflect, that Newman took so negative an attitude to Hopkins's well-meant suggestion, with the result that we will never know the poet's ideas on the psychology of religious assent! All the same, we may further reflect, on comparing Newman's treatise with Hopkins's writings in poetry and prose, it may not be so difficult for us to conjecture the main lines of Hopkins's proposed commentary. And that is what I now propose to attempt.

From the outset it may be remarked that common to both men is not only the outward fact but also the inner psychology of conversion, which is so basic to their lives and writings. In the case of Newman, the historical process of his conversion to the Catholic Church, as the outcome of his role in the Tractarian, or Oxford, Movement, is narrated in his *Apologia pro Vita Sua*, which he published in 1864. But the logical or psychological process of his motivation, culminating in his final assent to the Catholic Church—whose objective reasons he presented in his *Essay on the Development of Christian Doctrine* in the very year of his conversion, 1845—he went on to analyse in the seemingly impersonal terms of his *Grammar of Assent*, published in 1870.

As for Hopkins, his conversion to the Catholic Church, coming at a later stage of the Oxford Movement, may be seen as a direct result of his reading of Newman's recently published *Apologia*. It was no doubt for this reason that he specially requested Newman, whom he hadn't yet met in person, to receive him into the Catholic Church at the Oratory, Birmingham (of which Newman was in charge); and that accordingly took place in October 1866. Subsequently, we may trace his development of a personal and poetic analysis of his psychology of conversion in the poems from "The Wreck" onwards. Possibly it was his intention to offer this analysis in a more prosaic, objective, even argumentative form in his proposed commentary on Newman's book—only to find his hopes dashed by Newman's unwillingness to cooperate.

Turning now to this great poem of shipwreck, it was ostensibly composed on the occasion of the tragic wreck of the *Deutschland* at the mouth of the Thames in early December 1875 and of the drowning of some fifty passengers and crew, including five Franciscan nuns. At the same time, through this incident outside himself the poet looks back to a previous incident involving himself and his conversion a decade earlier. This is the point of the first part of the poem, to which the poet evidently turned after having composed the second part, thereby presenting his account of the shipwreck in the form of what he calls a Pindaric ode, but what we might also call (with echoes of Wordsworth) a lyrical ballad. As for the first part, it is clearly autobiographical in the romantic vein and strictly true of himself, as he declared to his friend Robert Bridges.

In this first part, the poet refers to the divine impact on his soul in terms of the sense of touch, or the inspiration of the Holy Spirit as finger of God: "Over again I feel thy finger and find thee"—where "over again" implies rebirth as what is nowadays called a "born again Christian". This rebirth is further described in stanza 2 in terms of a storm, with "lightning and lashed rod", in which the poet comes out with his impulsive assent to or confession of God's Word: "I did say yes." This is the occasion he subsequently recalls in his dark sonnet "Carrion Comfort", in speaking of "that night, that year/ Of now done darkness I wretch lay wrestling with (my God!) my God."

To what extent, it may now be asked, is Hopkins's analysis of religious assent in his poem as a whole indebted to Newman's earlier prosaic analysis in his *Grammar*? At least, we know that Hopkins read that book during his final year of philosophy at St. Mary's Hall, Stonyhurst, in 1873; and we may point to certain basic themes in it which are apparently taken up by the poet. Such, for instance, is the theme of divine providence, or what Hopkins calls in stanza 31 "lovely-felicitous Providence" and depicts in stanza 12 under the image of a mother bird brooding over her young "under thy feathers". This theme is notably emphasized by Newman in his *Grammar*, where he remarks that "what Scripture especially illustrates from its first page to its last is

God's Providence", adding that this "is nearly the only doctrine held with a real assent by the mass of religious Englishmen". He goes on to speak of a mind that has been "carefully formed upon the basis of its natural conscience", and so looks beyond the uniform laws of nature on the surface of the world (the sphere of physical science) to the hidden workings of a "particular Providence", in which it finds "the true key of that maze of vast complicated disorder". In the same way, Hopkins describes "the tall nun" in stanza 29, with her "heart right" and "single eye", reading "the unshapeable shock night" and knowing "the who and the why". Newman also speaks of "this instinct of the mind recognizing an external Master in the dictate of conscience", in words that seem to be recalled by Hopkins at the beginning of stanza 19: "Sister, a sister calling/ A master, her master and mine."

A second, related theme is that of the heart, which the poet mentions in stanza 18 as "mother of being in me, heart". Similarly, we find Newman typically declaring, "The heart is commonly reached, not through the reason, but through the imagination." Here we may recognize echoes of the well-known sayings of Shakespeare in his *Phoenix and the Turtle*, "Love hath reason, reason none", and of Pascal in his *Pensées*, "The heart has its reasons which the reason knows not." Newman also goes on to speak, in a continuation of the above-quoted passage on conscience, of "the theology of a religious imagination" as having "a living hold on truths which are really to be found in the world, though they are not upon the surface", and so gaining "a more and more consistent and luminous vision of God from the most unpromising materials". This vision is even described by Hopkins with reference to the nun in the culminating stanza 28 of his poem—or rather, it isn't so much described by him as conveyed to the reader in a series of abrupt breaks in the description, according to the figure of aposiopesis: "But how shall I . . . make me room there;/ Reach me a . . . Fancy, come faster!/ Strike you the sight of it? Look at it loom there,/ Thing that she . . . There then! the Master." It fully accords with Newman's characterization of the living thought of man, not least in the moment of conversion: "Thought is too keen and manifold, its sources are too remote and hidden, its paths too personal, delicate and circuitous, its subject-matter too various and intricate, to admit of the trammels of any language, of whatever subtlety and of whatever compass."

When, moreover, we turn from "The Wreck" to Hopkins's subsequent poems, we continue to find echoes of Newman's *Grammar* that deepen our appreciation of the other's influence and indicate the probable content of the poet's commentary. Almost at the beginning of the *Grammar* there occurs the charming picture of a child's mother teaching him "to repeat a passage from Shakespeare" and on his asking "the meaning of a particular line" her answering "that he was too young to understand it yet, but that . . . he would one day know". This is the picture to which Hopkins seems to recur in his "Spring and Fall", in which he imagines a little girl weeping over the falling leaves of autumn; and he comforts her with the words, "Now no matter, child, the name:/ Sorrow's springs are the same./ Nor mouth had, no nor mind, expressed/ What heart heard of, ghost guessed."

Also early on in his book Newman comments on the power of memory to reproduce such sense impressions as "the flavour of a peach as if it were in season . . . as of something individual". This is an idea and an image to which Hopkins frequently recurs in both his poems and his prose writings. The very image we find in "The Bugler's First Communion", where he speaks of the boy's "limber liquid youth, that to all I teach/ Yields tender as a pushed peach,/ Hies headstrong to its wellbeing of a self-wise self-will". Already in stanza 8 of "The Wreck" we find the similar image of "a lush-kept plush-capped sloe/ . . . mouthed to flesh-burst". Also in his commentary on the *Spiritual Exercises* of St. Ignatius, he vividly describes "that taste of myself, of I and me above and in all things, which is more distinctive than the taste of ale or alum, more distinctive than the smell of walnutleaf or camphor".

Here we touch upon that emphasis on eccentricity, individuality, and selfhood which is so basic to the poetic theory of Hopkins. This is what impresses us in such poems as "Pied Beauty", where the poet exults in "All things counter, original, spare, strange", and "As kingfishers catch fire", where he admires how "Each mortal thing does one thing and the same;/ . . . Selves—goes itself; *myself* it speaks and spells", and "To what serves Mortal Beauty?", where he emphasizes how "Self flashes off frame and face." The same emphasis is no less basic to Newman's *Grammar*, with his characteristic insistence that "words, which denote things, have innumerable implications", that units must "come first and (so-called) universals second", and that universals must "minister to units, not units be sacrificed to universals", also that "there is no such thing as stereotyped humanity". In Newman's insistence we may easily perceive his underlying criticism of the scholastic method, which would reduce all argument to "syllogistic reasoning", with each term starved down "till it has become the ghost of itself, and everywhere one and the same ghost, *'omnibus umbra locis'* . . . a notion neatly turned out of the laboratory of the mind, and sufficiently tame and subdued because existing only in a definition". It may even have been this criticism of the scholastic method that chiefly appealed to Hopkins, who had from the time of his philosophical studies at Stonyhurst turned for much the same reasons from the "universalism" of Aquinas and Suarez (and of Aristotle behind them) to the "individualism" of Scotus with his rare skill in the unraveling of "realty" (as he recalls it in "Duns Scotus's Oxford").

There still remains, for us to consider, an even deeper impact of Newman's *Grammar* on Hopkins's mind and poetry, as seen in his later, darker sonnets composed only a few years after his proposal of a commentary. For in the later pages of his *Grammar* we find Newman—as also in the later pages of his *Apologia*—turning to the themes of the hidden nature of God and his seeming absence from the created world. Thus in his dark sonnets the poet complains of "dark heaven's baffling ban" (in "To seem the stranger"); he compares his laments to "cries countless, cries like dead letters sent/ To dearest him that lives alas! Away" (in "I wake and feel"); he asks, "Where is he who more and more distils/ Delicious kindness?" and answers, "He is patient" (in "Patience, hard thing!")—as if exhorting himself to a similar patience.

All the poet can do in his sad situation is, it seems, to suffer. But then he might have drawn comfort from Newman's words, "We all suffer for each other and gain by each other's sufferings." What Hopkins gained from his own and no doubt from Newman's similar sufferings, not to mention the physical sufferings of the five nuns on the *Deutschland*, was his unique contribution to the second spring of the Catholic Church in England and elsewhere—a contribution that came to appear and to flower only in the second half of the twentieth century.

(*Hopkins Research* 29, December 2000)

Finding God in Hopkins

UNQUESTIONABLY one of the themes dearest to the heart of St. Ignatius is that of "finding God in all things". But what precisely does he mean by this expression? I would say he has two meanings in mind, or rather he uses two verbs with more or less the same meaning. One is the verb "seek", as used in one of the rules of the old "Summary of the Constitutions": *"In omnibus quaerant Deum"*—Let them seek God in all things. The other is the verb "find", as the outcome of seeking. Naturally we think that "seek" ought to come first, and then we may "find": the former ought to precede the latter. But the great St. Augustine isn't so sure. From the outset of his *Confessions* he puzzles over this problem, whether seeking comes first or finding. For, he says, when we seek God, it is a sign that we have already found him. As for myself, in most of the passages I have come across with these expressions, whether in the *Exercises* or the Constitutions, I find that St. Ignatius puts the seeking of God first, with emphasis on the will of God; whereas in most books I have read on Ignatian spirituality I find more emphasis on the importance of finding God in all things.

I think it may be said, to begin with, that St. Ignatius is nothing if not practical. He wants us to be ever seeking to *do* the will of God, to fix our minds on that one aim, to renounce and mortify ourselves and our personal inclinations. He seems to distrust any form of mystical vision, such as we find implied in a third verb, which is used more often by Father Jerome Nadal than by St. Ignatius, namely, "seeing" God in all things. Yet it is this third verb which I find most characteristic of the Ignatian spirituality in the poems of Hopkins. So now let me consider these three verbs, "seek", "find", and "see", as all claiming their rightful place in one and the same expression of the Jesuit ideal. It isn't, I submit, so much a question as to which of the three is the most Ignatian. That would be too invidious. It is rather a question as to how they are to be distinguished from each other. One might say that the three verbs are variously indicative of three stages in what St. Ignatius also calls "familiarity with God". First, one has to seek God in all things. Then, one comes to find him in them. Lastly, one sees in them a kind of anticipation of the beatific vision in heaven, such as that St. Ignatius himself beheld on the banks of the river Cardoner near Manresa—and in later life he could recapture that moment whenever he knelt down to pray in his room in Rome.

This memory may be illustrated by an episode related by Father Jerome Nadal, where he says of St. Ignatius: "He was lifted up by anything whatsoever, as happened, for example, one day I was with him in the garden, and looking at a leaf of an orange tree, he went into a lofty, elevated discourse about the Trinity." Such a passage of "seeing" God in a leaf of an orange tree we hardly expect to find in the *Exercises* or the Constitutions, being as it is of such an intimate nature. Yet it is amply borne out by what Father Joseph Conwell says of the saint in his book *Contemplation in Action*: "What is striking about the life of Ignatius is not so much his genius for organization as his complete immersion in the supernatural, his awareness of the supernatural, his awareness of the supernatural context of all things." Then he goes on to say about Father Nadal: "It is this that Nadal places as the ideal for every Jesuit: to look upon all things as new, completely changed, profounder in meaning, richer in significance, because seen in the fullness of their reality as creatures issuing from the Triune God." Only he adds an important caution, that such a grasp "of the Trinity-pervaded universe is not merely a vision, a wonderment, an awe, an overwhelming gasp at the beauty and magnificence and grandeur of it all: it is an immensely practical surging forward to meet and tangle with a world in revolt against that beauty and grandeur and love."

This may all serve as prelude to a deeper discussion on the poetry of Hopkins. For Father Conwell's words about "beauty and grandeur and love" come straight out of that poetry, though he never so much as once mentions the name of Hopkins in his book. After all, which poem of Hopkins do his words evoke so literally as the sonnet on "God's Grandeur", with its impressive opening line, "The world is charged with the grandeur of God"? What is more, the sonnet concludes with the Ignatian vision of "the Holy Ghost" brooding "over the bent world . . . with warm breast and with ah! bright wings". This may recall another saying of Father Nadal about the prayer of St. Ignatius, who "held intercourse with the divine persons and found a variety of gifts from the different persons but in this contemplation he found greater gifts in the person of the Holy Spirit".

Still, one may ask, isn't Hopkins in this poem merely indulging in a mystical vision of the world, without tangling (as Father Conwell puts it) "with a world in revolt"? Not at all, so long as we read his poem as a whole and not just in part. For if he stands in awe at "the grandeur of God" in the world, he is no less appalled at the obtuseness of men who "now not reck his rod", who sear all "with trade", who blear, smear all "with toil", who impress on all their "smudge" and "smell". Yet, he continues, "for all this nature is never spent;/ There lives the dearest freshness deep down things." And this freshness he attributes, with the eyes of faith, to the indwelling presence of the Holy Spirit.

This reminds me of a dispute I once had in London with a certain Columban priest, who often speaks and writes with fervour on the environmental problem, as he has experienced it in the Philippines. In the course of our dispute, in the presence of a Catholic publisher, who had (I suspect) mischievously pitted us together like fighting cocks, I maintained, with Hopkins, that "there lives the dearest freshness deep down things", and that somehow, for all the damage done by "dear and dogged man", as Hopkins characterizes the culprit, things will come out all right in the long run. Both in the world of nature and in the world of man, not to mention the world of the present-day Church, we must have faith and hope, even against hope, in the continued brooding of the Holy Spirit "over the bent world". But the Columban, for all my professed sympathy with him in his basic stand on the environment, couldn't accept my faith or my hope. He insisted on immediate action. But what action could we take, two weak individuals in a world at war? What was the point of our calling for action at once, when no one would listen to our words? As we say, there's no point in beating one's head against a brick wall. The head is more likely to suffer than the wall.

Anyhow, let me now go to the greatest, the longest, and the most Ignatian of Hopkins's poems, "The Wreck of the Deutschland". In it he most vividly expresses the outcome of his seven years of Jesuit formation, which were also years of "elected silence", on the occasion of a shipwreck at the mouth of the Thames, involving the tragic drowning of five Franciscan nuns. He typically begins his poem of thirty-five stanzas with a prayer to God, "Thou mastering me,/God", and at the end of the first stanza he hails the Holy Spirit, the "finger of God's right hand" (from the hymn *Veni Creator Spiritus*): "Over again I feel thy finger and find thee"— with stresses on each of those last two words.

Once again, it seems as if the poet is content to remain lost in contemplation, as he admires the action of God in the world, and even kisses his hand to the stars, "lovely asunder/ Starlight, wafting him out of it". He delights to recognize the presence of God "under the world's splendour and wonder" and lays stress on the mystery, as "I greet him the days I meet him, and bless when I understand." Yet the appeal of the mystery is, as he realizes, "tenderer in prayer apart"; while his present insistence is, after the model of St. Ignatius, on the need of coming to grips with the problem of the drowning nuns. With them, amid their dense and driven passion on board the foundering ship, the poet looks with the eyes of faith to the "feathery delicacy" of the "lovely-felicitous" providence of the Father, the condescending mercy of "the Christ of the Father compassionate", and the brooding wings of the Holy Spirit, bringing to completion the hidden presence of the "three-numbered form" of God.

Again and again this is the pattern of the poet's thought and prayer. Almost every poem of his, or at least several poems taken together, serves to bring out this contrast between God as above and in all the works of nature and "man, proud man, most ignorant of what he's most assured, his glassy essence" (as Isabella exclaims in Shakespeare's

Measure for Measure). Two poems in particular must be quoted in this context, since more than others they reveal Hopkins as an ecological prophet. In each case, the poet is weeping over what man has done in his blind folly to the beauty of nature. In "Binsey Poplars" he speaks so tenderly of these trees lining the river at Binsey near Oxford, as "My aspens dear, whose airy cages quelled,/ Quelled or quenched in leaves the leaping sun,/ All felled, felled, are all felled." We can almost hear the sobbing in his voice, as he registers his protest against the men responsible, for whatever reason, for this destruction of the inscapes of nature. Again, in "Ribblesdale", a lovely Lancashire valley near the Jesuit college of Stonyhurst, he expresses poetic sympathy for "Earth, sweet Earth, sweet landscape", against the selfishness of "dear and dogged man" who is "to his own selfbent so bound, so tied to his turn". Such sympathy is all too often dismissed by hard-headed moderns as "pathetic fallacy"; but it is rather the critics who are falsely insisting on a rigid separation between man and nature, to the prejudice of both nature and eventually man.

That isn't all there is to be said concerning the Ignatian prayer and mystical vision of Hopkins. What he sees outside himself in the world—recalling what Newman, too, in his *Apologia*, saw as "a sight which fills me with unspeakable distress"—Hopkins comes to see also within himself in his dark sonnets. Here what we find is no longer the presence but the absence of God, as the poet utters, with the unspeakable groanings which St. Paul attributes to the Holy Spirit, "cries like dead letters sent/ To dearest him that lives alas! away". In another of these sonnets he asks, "And where is he who more and more distils/ Delicious kindness?"—only to receive the answer, "He is patient." As Christ himself is said to have reassured St. Teresa on a similar occasion,

God is present even in his absence, or then especially by means of the precious virtue of patience. After all, suffering isn't so much a metaphysical problem for the minds of theologians as a practical solution to the greater problem of evil, a solution that God himself inflicts on sinful men, including saints, for our greater good and instruction.

Such is Hopkins's poetic commentary on the teaching of St. Ignatius, which is to be found not so much in the Constitutions as in the *Exercises*, notably in the final "Contemplation for the Obtaining of Divine Love". It is here, above all, that St. Ignatius, after having led the exercitant through the several stages of "seeking" and "finding" God in all things, brings him to the final stage of "seeing" God as present in all things and as working through them, till everything good is seen as descending from above, like rays from the sun or waters from a fountain. And it is here, I may add, that St. Ignatius is joined by those two great English poets, not only Hopkins but also Shakespeare, in a single Trinitarian vision of divine love. So I may fitly conclude with Hopkins's words on this contemplation: "All things therefore are charged with love, are charged with God, and if we know how to touch them give off sparks and take fire, yield drops and flow, ring and tell of him." Such, too, is the life commended by Shakespeare in *As You Like It*, which "Finds tongues in trees, books in the running brooks,/ Sermons in stones, and good in everything."

(*Hopkins Research* 30, December 2001)

The Self as Other in Hopkins

For my text let me take three of the sonnets composed by Hopkins at Dublin during his dark year of 1885: first, "To seem the stranger"; secondly, "I wake and feel"; and lastly, "My own heart". Now let me go back to what Shakespeare calls "the dark backward and abysm of time", to the boyhood years of Hopkins, following what he calls not just "hours" but "years" and even "life". I refer to the age of adolescence when, as Wordsworth says, "shades of the prison-house begin to close/ Upon the growing boy". For this I have no hard evidence to offer, only the fact that a precocious boy such as Hopkins, outstanding not only in his studies but also in a talent for poetry, but less so on the playing fields, must have been looked at askance by not a few of his classmates and even his teachers. Boys can be so cruel to one another! With his growing intellect, such a boy is more than ordinarily aware of himself and correspondingly cut off from his fellows—which brings him to that contrast between the Self and the Other which plays so large a part in the development both of his personality and of his poetry.

In a sense, the whole of Hopkins's life as a person and a poet may be seen in terms of a search for Self, partly by means of, partly at the expense of the Other. This is what inclined him at Oxford to become one of a close circle of intimate friends at Balliol College, those who were likeminded with him in intellectual, poetic, and above all religious interests. This was what drew him to the remnants of the old Oxford Movement under the direction of Edward Pusey and Henry Liddon and to read with excited attention the pages of Newman's *Apologia pro Vita Sua* soon after it was published in 1864. This was what introduced him not only to the thought of "two luminous beings, myself and God", but also to his disillusionment in the Anglican Church as a "half-way house", not a true home for his restless spirit. So he left his family, friends, and even studies behind him, in order to be received into the Catholic Church by Newman himself at Birmingham. Then, with Newman's approval, he went a step further and joined the Society of Jesus at Manresa House, Roehampton.

No wonder Hopkins came to seem a stranger in the eyes of almost everyone; for he had cut himself off from almost everyone he had known—family, friends, and countrymen—in his search for those two luminous beings of Newman, himself and God. In order to become himself and so to find God, or rather, to lose himself and so find himself in God, or as Coleridge puts it, in order to "proceed from the self in order to lose and find all self in God", Hopkins renounced his connections with the Other, with the inhabitants of the outside world, in his interpretation of the call of Christ the King as presented by St. Ignatius in the *Spiritual Exercises*, "to act against one's own sensuality, one's carnal and worldly love", even including the love of family, friends, and countrymen, to be detached from all things and persons in order to follow Jesus Christ and him alone.

The poetry of Hopkins, too, was included in this act of self-abnegation, in the form of what he subsequently regretted as a "massacre of the innocents", when he decided to impose on himself—without taking the advice of another—a rule of "elected silence". So when he later felt freed by a wise suggestion of his rector at St. Beuno's College to return to the composition of poetry, he began his new poem, "The Wreck of the Deutschland", with the old Newmanian, new Ignatian, juxtaposition of "Thou mastering me,/ God." He also went on to speak of a mysterious moment of spiritual struggle when, like Jacob wrestling with the angel, he felt himself overwhelmed by the divine power and "I did say yes/ O at lightning and lashed rod". Was this, we may wonder, the moment of his conversion at Oxford from the Anglican to the Catholic Church under Newman's influence? Or was it the other moment of his conversion to a dedicated religious life as a Jesuit under the influence of St. Ignatius, owing to a retreat he made under Jesuit direction at that time? Or was it perhaps a "golden thread" in his life leading him, like Newman, from moment to moment of successive conversions in a gradual purification of his lower human self to union with the supreme Self, or I AM, of God?

One thing we notice in the succession of bright sonnets composed by Hopkins in the aftermath of "The Wreck" is a new insistence on self, the new self he has discovered by his rejection of his old self, in contrast to "the Other", or "what man has made of man" in the outside world. This is also Newmanian, as Newman describes it in his *Apologia*, how after starting "with the being of a God" he looks out of himself "into the world of men" and there sees "a sight which fills me with unspeakable distress". Already in "The Wreck" we note how readily the poet speaks to himself, as "My heart, but you were dove-winged, I can tell", and as "mother of being in me, heart". At the same time, he can never forget "the Other", not with rejection but with compassion, as he feels "pity of the rest of them", those others involved with the five nuns in the shipwreck—somewhat like Miranda in Shakespeare's *Tempest*. From them he has turned away in his resolution to devote himself to Christ in religious life as a Jesuit; but that was only to turn back to them all the more effectively after his years of religious formation. He has had to lose himself and all else in order to find himself in union with Christ, not for his own sake, but to help others to find their true selves in the same union with Christ.

A notable example of this new concern of Hopkins comes in the first of his bright sonnets, "God's Grandeur". Here we find him not only, as he puts it in his translation of St. Thomas's Latin hymn *Adoro Te Devote*, "Lost, all lost in wonder at the God thou art"—the God whose grandeur is everywhere present "under the world's splendour and wonder"—but also filled with grief that men "now not reck his rod". This contrast comes up everywhere, not just in the opposition between the reformed self of the poet and the unreformed selves of men in the outside world. Rather, when he feels tempted to make such an opposition in "The Candle Indoors", Hopkins suddenly, even bewilderingly, rounds on himself with the indignant rebuke, "Come you indoors, come home!" and "Are you beam-blind, yet to a fault/ In a neighbour deft-handed?" Rather, the opposition as he sees it is between the world of nature, as created by God and still retaining vestiges of his creative presence everywhere, and the world of men, who are even now in the industrial age treading all things underfoot, searing all with their nasty smudge and smell. Such is his lament, a strangely prophetic, ecological lament, for the recently felled trees in "Binsey Poplars" and for the Earth itself, "sweet Earth, sweet landscape", in "Ribblesdale". It is all the handiwork, all the responsibility of him whom he describes as "dear and dogged man", who is at once "the heir" to the kingdom of heaven and yet "To his own self-bent so bound, so tied to his turn".

So long as Hopkins was living his Jesuit life in seclusion from "the world", so long as he was pursuing his philosophical and theological studies in his Jesuit formation at St. Mary's Hall, Stonyhurst, and at St. Beuno's College, he could see all this from a distance and shake his head over it, while maintaining his joy in "the grandeur of God". But once he left that formation and was sent as a priest into the world in a succession of temporary tasks, at Farm Street church in London, at St. Aloysius's church in Oxford, at St. Joseph's church in Bedford Leigh, at St. Francis Xavier's church in Liverpool, at another church of St. Joseph in Glasgow, he came to see—as Newman had already seen it at his Oratory in Birmingham—all the misery of the lower classes in the Victorian industrial age from close up. And that was a sight which filled him, as it had filled Newman, "with unspeakable distress". From time to time it might fill him with a paradoxical comfort, as in his brief acquaintance with the dying "Felix Randal"; but even that comfort was not unmixed with tears of anguish.

The climax to all this came when Hopkins was sent by his provincial superior, not as a priest but as a professor, to the re-established University College founded some thirty years before by Newman in Dublin. It was a climax in the sense of a crescendo of grief, as "More pangs will, schooled at forepangs, wilder wring"—a grief in which the poet can find no comfort, whether from the Holy Spirit, "the Comforter", or from "Mary, mother of us". For now he feels more cut off than ever before, not only from family and friends, but also from "England, whose honour O all my heart woos, wife/ To my creating thought". Now he isn't even a priest, as when he could tend to the spiritual needs of the faithful in industrial cities, but a mere university teacher, involved more in the weary task of correcting examinations than in the more rewarding task of giving lectures. Now he is "at a third remove" from his English home; now he is in a land "where wars are rife", wars against his own country and countrymen. Now he hasn't even the comforting presence of friends who can appreciate his poems; nor can he get them printed and divulged to "the yet unknowing world". Now he can only hoard them without getting them any hearing; or if he can find friends to hear them through the medium of correspondence, such friends as Bridges only seem to criticize them and so leave them unheard. And so the poor poet is left "a lonely began". With all his priestly and religious formation, he has been sent by his superiors, standing for him in the place of Christ, into the world, and like Christ, he hasn't been received by the world. Accordingly he feels all the abandonment of Christ on the cross, as expressed in the cry, "My God, my God, why hast thou abandoned me?"

No wonder Hopkins awakes in the early hours one day in Dublin in 1885, feeling "the fell of dark, not day". No wonder he looks back not just over "the black hours" he has spent alone with his heart during the night, but over all the years of his past Jesuit life, his series of religious conversions, his life as a whole. All this time he has devoted himself to the cause of God; and for this he is rejected not just by the world (which would be understandable) but by God himself. As he complains in the spirit of Job and Jeremiah in a later sonnet, "Oh, the sots and thralls of lust/ Do in spare hours more thrive than I that spend,/ Sir, life upon thy cause." For God he has given up everything; but from God he has received nothing, but only abandonment. "Wert thou mine enemy", he complains, "O thou my friend"—with echoes of a similar complaint made by St. Teresa of Avila to Christ—"How would'st thou worst, I wonder than thou dost/ Defeat, thwart me?" He is nothing if not frank and straightforward, even downright rude, with God!

Now we come to the climax within the climax, or rather the anti-climax within the anti-climax of complaint, as within the pitchblack darkness of his "dark night of the soul" Hopkins cuts a dividing cleft not only between himself and the outside world, but within layer upon layer of himself. Now he feels himself paradoxically "other" to himself. In denying himself to follow Christ as his true self, he has found himself divided from himself. Nor is it just the unreceptive outside world that is rejecting him and dividing him from himself, but he is himself dividing himself from himself. Or as he himself puts it in the third of the texts we are considering, he is living "this tormented mind/ With this tormented mind tormenting yet". Here is the poor poet, tormenting himself; and the means with which he is tormenting himself is "this tormented mind". Here in another sense from which he has spoken of himself as being "at a third remove" from his family, his friends, and his countrymen, he is at a remove from his inmost self. He is one self, as subject; and he is engaged in tormenting himself, as object, by means of his tormented mind, as agent. One after another, his selves are all occupied in an inner circle of self-torment, as it were an inner circle of hell, and this leads him to recognize, "The lost are like this, and their scourge to be/ As I am mine their sweating selves; but worse."

In other words, the poet is indulging in a paroxysm of self-pity, which he evidently knows is morally wrong even in his words of self-exhortation, "My own heart let me more have pity on." It is a strangely paradoxical situation, in which he wishes to show more pity on his heart by indulging less in self-pity. For in such a situation, when a person is preoccupied with thoughts of self-pity, the only advice one can give him is, "Forget about yourself! Go for a walk! Do something so as to occupy your mind with something else!" And that is how Hopkins advises himself in this poem, speaking to himself as he might be giving counsel to another in the same situation: "Come, poor Jackself, I do advise/ You, jaded, let be; call off thoughts awhile/ Elsewhere: leave comfort rootroom." If he is always thinking about himself, worrying about himself, indulging in pity for himself, how can he expect God to come to him bringing words of comfort, smiling "as skies/ Betweenpie mountains"? Then he may expect, as he finds in his later poem, "That Nature is a Heraclitean Fire", to see the divine light of comfort as "A beacon, an eternal beam" shining across his "foundering deck" and directing his eyes from his feeling of abandonment on the cross to his hope in the resurrection of Christ.

All this process of loss and gain, of conversion and rejection, we may interpret, if we like, in medical terms of chronic ill-health, exacerbated by his Irish exile, or in Freudian, psychological terms of maladjustment to his contemporary world and to his own psychic condition, or in biographical terms of the depressing air of Dublin and of work for which he was illsuited being loaded on his shoulders, or in mystical terms of a "dark night of the soul", which he had to undergo for the further purification of his soul according to the inscrutable designs of divine providence. But for my present purpose it is enough to attribute the process to an intricate interweaving of the self and the other in the deeply concerned mind of Hopkins. At the same time, it may be presented in terms of his Victorian age, which was absorbed, more than any preceding age in human history, in preoccupation with the self.

In particular, we may see this as no small part of Newman's influence on Hopkins; and yet it was also deeply operative in the influence of St. Ignatius, whose whole aim in his *Exercises* is to bring the exercitant face to face with himself, so as to ask himself, "Who am I?" and then face to face with God, so as to ask him the further question, "Who art thou?" Newman himself may, of course, have learnt this twofold question from St. Ignatius, already from his Anglican years. Or he may have learnt it from Descartes, with his famous dictum, "I think; therefore I am"—not overlooking, what most people overlook, the subsequent proof Descartes offers for the existence of God based on the famous ontological argument of St. Anselm. In this way, already before Newman, it may be said that for Descartes, too, there were "two luminous beings", himself and God. Unfortunately, Descartes all too soon forgot about God's existence in his concern to prove the existence of the outside world, or the "other". Yet from him has come so much in modern philosophy, not least the German philosophy from Kant and Fichte onwards, with its growing preoccupation with the transcendental Self.

But now I have let myself be distracted from the spiritual process in Hopkins, by looking away from his own self-description in poetic terms to the various conflicting influences at work in the world of his time. It may indeed be good to pay some attention to them, as it may be good to pay some attention to the medical, psychological, and biographical terms mentioned above. But it is always necessary to come back to the poet himself and his poems, in which the interrelations between the Self and the Other are continually crossing and criss-crossing in endlessly repeated and variegated patterns. At the same time, I am irresistibly reminded not only of Newman or St. Ignatius or Duns

Scotus (whom I haven't yet mentioned), but also of Shakespeare, with his intertwining of "To be" and "not to be", or "I am" and "nothing", or the merely human "I am" and the divine "I AM".

(*Hopkins Research* 31, December 2002)

The Eccentricity of Hopkins

THE ODDITY or eccentricity of Hopkins is a commonplace of criticism concerning his poems even from the time he sent manuscripts of them to his Oxford friend Robert Bridges. In their correspondence we find Hopkins now defending himself from his friend's criticism, now apologizing to him and resolving to do better in the future. But to what extent, may we ask, was he justified in his admitted oddity or eccentricity, and to what extent was his friend justified in his criticisms?

First, we have to realize how eccentric Hopkins was in an age and nation of eccentrics. There can surely be few nations in the world so eccentric, or so proud of their eccentricity, as the English, notably in the Victorian age. And here is Hopkins appearing in the very midst of this age, with the dates of both his birth and his death falling well within the reign of Queen Victoria. The more we examine the early years of Hopkins during his poetic formation, the more we find him heading in the direction of eventual eccentricity. Brought up within an artistic and musical middle-class family in North London, he was, we find, already something of a rebel at school—as he had good cause to be. On the strength of a classical scholarship he went up to Balliol College, Oxford;

and during his studies there we find him fascinated with the eccentric philosophy of the Greek philosopher Parmenides and the eccentric art criticism of John Ruskin. From these two mentors, classical and contemporary, in philosophy and art, he derived much of his later professed taste for the individual, the unique, the eccentric, including his first references to his favourite ideas of "inscape" and "instress".

The same cult of eccentricity we may see at work in his conversion to the Catholic Church, while still an undergraduate student at Oxford, when he journeyed to Birmingham in order to be received into the Church by that other Victorian eccentric, John Henry Newman. Possibly the strangest event in this history of eccentricity took place when Hopkins decided, unlike Newman, though with Newman's encouragement, to enter the strict religious order of the Jesuits, whose regimen might seem calculated to quench all sparks of originality and eccentricity in their members during their long years of formation. Yet it was apparently with Hopkins, as with the daisies of the field, that the more he was trodden underfoot in the interests of humility and mortification, the more his eccentricity multiplied and flourished, till it came to full fruition in his poem on "The Wreck of the Deutschland", with the approval of the rector at St. Beuno's College.

Everything about this poem has the outward appearance of conventionality: the form of a Pindaric ode, combined with that of a lyrical ballad; the composition in stanzas of eight lines each, with a regular rhyme scheme and a regular rhythm maintained throughout its thirty-five stanzas. So much for the outward appearances. Yet within the substance of the poem, everything—for all these self-imposed restrictions—is designed to break out of such convention with revolutionary power. The poem is, it may be said, nothing if not eccentric. So we may well forgive the poor Jesuit editor of *The Month*, though a personal friend of the poet, for judging that his Victorian readers weren't yet ready for such strong wine.

From the outset what is evident about this new poem is the strong, even violent, beat of its rhythm, which the poet chose to term "sprung". "Thou mastering me,/ God . . ./ Over again I feel thy finger and find thee." What strength, what spring, what splendour there is in these two lines, opening and closing the first stanza! And what superb disregard of the conventionality of the standard "running rhythm"! Here we see a new poet, not so much singing to the charmed ears of his readers, or even speaking to them, as addressing God in an insistent, dramatic tone of voice, the like of which had hardly been heard of in English poetry since the days of William Shakespeare and John Donne! Then, we hear the alliteration, going with the stresses in each line, that had hardly been heard of in English poetry since the days of William Langland, to whose example in *Pierce Ploughman [sic]* the poet appeals in his Author's Preface— what with "lightning and lashed rod", "truer than tongue" and "terror", "walls, altar and hour", "a horror of height", "leaning of, laced with", all converging in the second stanza. Here are the unmistakable accents of a new revolutionary poet, bringing into the staid Victorian English a revival of Old English and an infusion of Welsh poetry.

What is even more notably eccentric about this poem, however, is the way the poet has deliberately tortured the grammar and syntax of his mother tongue—though not his ancestral tongue, insofar as his family origins were Welsh. And yet more notably eccentric are many of the rhymes, in which he merely seems to be kowtowing to contemporary convention, while harking back to Old English for his alliterative and stress metre. Thus all unexpectedly, in stanza 14, we come upon such rhymes as "leeward", "drew her/ D-", and "endured"; and subsequently, in stanza 31, such other rhymes as "Providence" with "of it, and/ S-". Such eccentric rhymes we may recognize from Byron's *Don Juan*, where the effect is deliberately one of burlesque. But here the poet's intention is hardly a comic one, except in the Shakespearian sense of comedy used to underline subsequent tragedy by the very contrast. Then, even more notably eccentric is the deep theological undercurrent in this elegiac ode— I mean, the way the Jesuit poet flies in the face of the contemporary aesthetic orthodoxy of "art for art's sake" in proposing an art for the combined sake of morality and theology. What, in heaven's name, his Victorian readers would have demanded, had they been given the chance of reading and judging the poem, has all this theology got to do with poetry? Even John Milton, for all his bare-faced and roundheaded Puritanism, would hardly (we think) have put such brazen scholastic theology into his *Paradise Lost*! (Yet he did.)

For all his eccentricity, however, Hopkins is impenitent—even when charged with it by his friend Robert Bridges. This is all no accident, as it were flung out in the excess of poetic inspiration. It is his very theory of poetry, developed by him in the school partly of St. Ignatius, partly of Duns Scotus. From the former he had learned to "find God in all things", and from the latter to respect the individuality, the this-ness of things, namely, that in them by which they are what they are. For him this wasn't just theology or spirituality or philosophy: It was poetry. And this aspect of poetry, this basic aspect of all poetry, he went on to brandish in the faces of his poetic readers, those privileged few who happened to be his correspondents, in his two poems, "Pied Beauty" and "As kingfishers catch fire".

The former poem may well be described as a bare-faced theological treatise, beginning with "Glory be to God" and ending with "Praise him"—as it were a typical Jesuit exercise beginning with the Ignatian motto, *"Ad Majorem Dei Gloriam"*, and ending with the other motto, *"Laus Deo Semper"*. Yet it is no conventional poem of divine praise, such as might be sung to a hymn tune in church. It is, like almost everything else in Hopkins's poetic oeuvre, a revolutionary poem, with special attention paid to "All things counter, original, spare, strange;/ Whatever is fickle, freckled (who knows how?)/ With swift, slow; sweet, sour; adazzle, dim". It seems as if the poet is commending his own eccentricity, oddity and originality, as seen in all the things around him with his eccentric, odd, and original eyes. Nor is it only that. He even has the temerity to attribute it all, with all its eccentricity, to God. After all, who—he wonders—originated the tyrannosaurus, the coelacanth, the behemoth, the alligator, the whale, the human being, but God, as though taking delight in all this comic, cock-eyed variety—as in fact we see him doing in Proverbs 8 and Job 39–41?

As for "kingfishers", it is Hopkins's theory of poetry in poetic form, with barely disguised acknowledgment to him who "of all men most sways my spirits to peace", Duns Scotus, whom he further praises as "Of realty the rarest-veined unraveller". What he seeks to do in all his poems is but to assist, in his humanity, "each mortal thing" to do what it does, namely, "one thing and the same", to deal out "that being indoors each one dwells", to self, to go itself, to speak and spell "myself". In this respect he is, as he says in "Ribblesdale", the eye, tongue, and heart of Earth, lending Earth his poetic "tongue to plead", his poetic "heart to feel"; while at the same time he expresses himself and fulfils himself as a theological, philosophical, eccentric poet. Or rather, what is specially eccentric in him is that he aims not merely at expressing himself (like another Milton) or things in the world around him (like another Wordsworth) but even the supreme SELF of God, as Father, Son, and Holy Spirit. He is not the end of his own poetry; but as combined poet and prophet, again not unlike Milton and Wordsworth, he feels himself the mouthpiece of God, even when he speaks to God as in the opening stanza of "The Wreck of the Deutschland". It is as if behind all his poetic output one may hear the words of Shakespeare's John of Gaunt in *Richard II*, "Methinks I am a prophet new inspired." He is indeed a prophet, arising paradoxically and unexpectedly out of an age notorious for its conventionality, while proclaiming revolution to a yet unborn modern age.

Not but what, we are constrained to add, he sought to appease his critical friend Robert Bridges, and even to apologize for his oddity, by writing poems which are in his opinion more restrained, classical, and Miltonic. Yet when we peruse these poems, which oddly satisfied Bridges, we can't help wondering at the oddity of Hopkins's idea of restraint. Take his other poem of shipwreck, "The Loss of the Eurydice", which Bridges oddly regarded as an improvement on "The Wreck of the Deutschland". It might well be included in any anthology of eccentric poems in English literature. If ever there was an eccentric poem, it is surely this, with its succession of odd rhymes that quite overshadow the two odd rhymes I have quoted from "The Wreck". Thus, it has "fully, on" rhyming with "bullion", "seamen" with "be men", "wrecked her? He/ C-" with "electric", "England" with "mingle? And", "portholes" with "mortals", "captain" with "wrapped in", "beach her" with "feature", "coast or/ M-" with "snowstorm", "suit! He" with "beauty", "busy to/ D-" with "visited", "crew, in" with "ruin". How, we may well wonder, can such comic burlesque go with the tragic theme of the poem—unless the poet has, for his own theological reasons, refused to take the tragedy seriously?

Then, we may take the more charming "Spring and Fall"—more charming in that it is supposedly addressed "to a young child". It was no doubt thanks to the constant criticism of his friend Bridges that Hopkins availed himself of this expedient to compose a simpler kind of poem, since the child was, he confessed, an invention of his Muse. To begin with, it does have an air of simplicity; but Hopkins, being the person and the poet he was, couldn't keep up this air of simplicity for long. Like Shakespeare, he is nothing if not complicated. And sure enough, before long the complication comes to the fore in such words as "worlds of wanwood leafmeal". Nor is that a merely poetic expression, but the thought also follows suit, leaving the poor child in a state, if she existed, of utter bewilderment. "Now no matter, child, the name", he reassures her, "Sorrow's springs are the same." And so he proceeds to conclude his reassurance with words that have left not only children but mature adult commentators perplexed to this day.

Further, we may take his "Andromeda", in which, he tells Bridges in his accompanying letter (to forestall the other's criticism), he has aimed "at a more Miltonic plainness and severity than I have anywhere else", so that it has come to appear to him "almost free from quaintness". Well, faced with such self-criticism, we can only exclaim, "If this is what Hopkins means by 'plainness', what can he possibly mean by 'obscurity'?" Again, if he thinks his poem is "free from quaintness", we can only assume he has a private meaning of "quaintness" not shared by his English readers. At least, for all his opening endeavour to put these qualities into his poem for the appeasement of his friend, once he has got under way, he can't help leaving himself and his words in the hands of his all too un-Miltonic Muse, culminating in such a quaint, complicated conclusion as: "All while her patience, morselled into pangs,/ Mounts; then to alight disarming, no one dreams,/ With Gorgon's gear and barebill/ thongs and fangs."

Not that I wish to criticize the poems of Hopkins with all their oddity and eccentricity. No, that is what I particularly admire in them. Without all this oddity and eccentricity he wouldn't have been Hopkins. And that goes even for the oddest of his odd rhymes in "The Loss of the Eurydice". Only, what he is, as Milton would say, "with all his singing robes about him", that is, in his poems, he is not in his prosaic commentary on his poems or in his feeble attempts to justify his seeming excesses in the face of Bridges's criticism. No, I say, there was no need for Hopkins to apologize for anything in his poems, whether to Bridges or to anyone else. They are what they are, works of poetic genius; and I wouldn't have them otherwise.

(*Hopkins Research* 31, December 2003)

Hopkins in Ireland

Poor Hopkins! We can't help feeling sympathy for him, caught as he was in the sad predicament he describes for us so poignantly in the "terrible sonnets" of his Dublin years. Surely there can be no poems in the whole compass of English literature that so painfully portray such agony as he feels in his Irish exile. It may all be seen as coming to a precisely defined climax in the sonnet "To seem the stranger".

Not only in the Dublin of 1885, but for almost as long as he can remember—for his agony isn't just a matter of hours or days, like the toothache, "but," he says, "where I say hours I mean years, mean life"—he has experienced the pain of "seeming the stranger" and of living his "life among strangers". From the time he was cut off from his warm family circle in Hampstead on going up to Oxford in 1863, and from the time he further cut himself off from the intellectual circle of his Oxford friends on his reception into the Catholic Church in 1866, and from the time he went on to enter the noviciate of the Society of Jesus at Manresa House, Roehampton, in 1868, he was moving more and more into an exile first of his own choosing, then at the discretion of his religious superiors, till he was sent by them across the Irish Sea to Dublin in 1884.

Now he finds himself "at a third remove" from his family, from his friends and acquaintances, even from his homeland, which he now hails as "wife to my creating thought". Here in Ireland he feels everything against him as never before, not only in his surroundings "where wars are rife", but even in himself, so as to make him "weary of idle a being". In Wales, at St. Beuno's College, he had been able to adjust himself to his foreign surroundings, partly because he was still with mainly English companions, partly because with his Welsh name of Hopkins he wasn't altogether a foreigner but was back in the land of his fathers. But in Ireland, at University College, he had little in common with the Irish around him, many of whom regarded him with hostility as an Englishman, while he for his part took no pains to hide his English identity.

Now, however, as if all this wasn't trouble enough for Hopkins, and more than enough to evoke our sympathy for him, along comes this unsympathetic biographer, Norman White, intent on knocking more metaphorical nails into the poet's coffin with his new study of *Hopkins in Ireland* (University College Dublin Press, 2002), as it were insulting over his lonely, anonymous grave in the cemetery of Glasnevin.

Already Hopkins has had more than his due share of unsympathetic biographers, who delight in driving a wedge between his priesthood and his poetry—a wedge for which Hopkins himself was partly to blame, owing to occasional words written in his letters to his family and friends. But now his latest biographer leaves us in doubt whether the poet wouldn't have been far better off if he had never become a Catholic or a Jesuit or a priest.

From White's all too jaundiced viewpoint, which he presses upon us again and again, what the poet found in his religion, in his religious order, and in his priesthood was next to nothing but "the limits of a narrow dogma", an unrelenting insistence of a didactic moralism, a "conformity to the correct ideological stance", a "moral straitjacket", the heavy obstacle of a "priestly philosophical framework", "a narrowly Victorian Manicheism", a set of "rigid intellectual schemata"—if I may range these repetitive phrases in the order they occur in the text.

Within such narrow limits and under such rigid supervision as the author is always imagining for us, one wonders how Hopkins was able to write poetry at all, let alone poetry of such surpassing excellence as is acknowledged by almost all literary critics—with the solitary exception of White.

How, one may further wonder, has White come to such an unfavourable conclusion, while advancing the claims of the artist over those of the religionist? "Art," he affirms, "could provide and succeed where religion had failed." He is speaking about the sonnet, "Thou art indeed just, Lord". Yet even here he is disappointed at "the stilted, derivative opening with Jeremiah, which provides a false start", owing (he surmises) to the rigid form of the religious retreat which the poet has just completed, preventing him from expressing and exorcizing "his intimate feelings". Also in the sonnet's conclusion he criticizes "the overdone alliterative harmony of the final line". All in all, he has hardly a good thing to say about this sonnet which he has put forward as an example of the triumph of art over religion!

Even in the earlier sonnet "Spelt from Sibyl's Leaves", to which he devotes a longer, more detailed analysis, White can't help contrasting the poet's foregoing expression of "nature's aesthetic qualities" with the way they are "nullified into black and white, and replaced by human ethical concerns". All he is able to appreciate in Hopkins is an aesthetic perception of natural beauty, but he is unable to follow the poet once the latter looks from the immediacy of nature to what White can only see and criticize as a moral didacticism. This is what White again and again rejects as "narrow". But it may be questioned whether the narrowness is in the mind of the poet or of the critic. As T. S. Eliot has said, in another context, "The corruption of the poet is the generation of the critic". Eliot is, of course, speaking of one individual like himself, first a poet and then a critic. But in the present case, one may say it is the critic who sees the poetry as corrupt, and it is his distortion of the poet that has made him so carping a critic, till hardly a poem of poor Hopkins is left unbleared, unsmeared with his critical toil.

From White's overwhelmingly critical viewpoint, wouldn't it have been better, one wonders, for Hopkins to have remained true to his poetic vocation, without subjecting his free mind to the petty trammels of the Catholic Church, the Society of Jesus, and his ultimate destination as a Jesuit in Ireland?

At least, we can see for ourselves the contrast between his earlier poems composed in his undergraduate days at Oxford and the later poems following on his seven years of "elected silence" after joining the noviciate of the Society of Jesus. It is the contrast between (say) "The Alchemist in the City", which in some ways looks forward to "The Windhover" with "my heart in hiding", and that supreme expression of Hopkins's genius, which he dedicated "To Christ our Lord" and which he described as "the best thing I ever wrote".

There are, I suppose, few critics who prefer the earlier poems to the later, in which almost all recognize a distinctive maturity of style. And that maturity is generally seen as achieved not in spite of but because of the intervening formation of the poet as a Jesuit and as a priest. Yet for some hidden reason, on which one can only speculate, it seems that White is incapable of admitting anything good or enriching or poetically formative in it.

Abstractly speaking, one assumes that as a scholar White has made the careful study of the Catholic Church and the Society of Jesus that is naturally expected of one who would venture to criticize the influence of those institutions on the mind of Hopkins. But when it comes down to concrete fact, his knowledge is patently defective, even to the extent of landing him in mistakes that may well be stigmatised as "schoolboy howlers".

Thus, concerning the Catholic Church, and following the order in which these errors occur in the text, White speaks of "the approved theologian Thomas Aquinas" as the "traditional opponent" of "the downgraded philosopher Duns Scotus"; whereas in fact it was Scotus who not only followed Aquinas but also went out of his way to oppose him—partly because Scotus was a Franciscan and Aquinas a Dominican. It may be true that Aquinas is generally "approved" in the Church, but Scotus has never been downgraded, least of all in his own Franciscan Order.

Next, White refers to the contrast drawn in "Spelt from Sibyl's Leaves" between "black, white; right, wrong", as originating in the old hymn *Dies Irae*, which isn't so very old as hymns go—only thirteenth century; whereas the contrast goes all the way back to the teaching of Christ and his apostles, if not to Moses. He then affirms that "in times of prosperity . . . the religious person believes that virtue will be rewarded on earth"; whereas that is by no means the teaching of Job or Jeremiah, let alone that of Christ himself. Their teaching may have been born in times of adversity, but it is still accepted by their followers in times of prosperity.

White goes on to dismiss what he calls "the weary plea for rest and mercy of the Agnus Dei", which prompts one to wonder if he has ever listened to a Gregorian chant of that triple invocation of Christ as Lamb of God at Mass. The weariness is surely all in the mind of the listener (if he has ever listened), not in that of the chanter. Then, he is so confident that "according to the theology of the time (Hopkins') family, as Protestants, could not enter Heaven after death"; but that is hardly the theology we find in the poems on "The Wreck" or "The Loss of the Eurydice", let alone "Henry Purcell".

Again, White speaks so oddly of "Aquinas's prescription that hope is the opposite of despair", which may be compared to a spurious appeal to Aristotle for the common saying that "Honesty is the best policy". He goes on to mention "Christian authorities" (whom he prudently refrains from naming) as responsible for allegorising "the epithalamic Song of Solomon into unsympathetic Christian contexts before its inclusion in the Bible", whereas it had been the Jewish authorities who first included that book in their canon of the Bible long before the Christians drew up their canon.

As for the attitude of the Society of Jesus to Hopkins's poems, White seems so sure that Hopkins's religious superiors disapproved of the poems—on the slender basis, to which he keeps on returning, that "The Wreck of the Deutschland" (which the poet had written at the express suggestion of his rector at St. Beuno's) was turned down by the editor of the Jesuit periodical *The Month*, Father Henry Coleridge, who happens to have been a good friend of Hopkins. White is adamant that this judgment—incidentally shared by Hopkins's poetic friend from Oxford days, Robert Bridges—represents an "official rejection" by the Society of Jesus; whereas few Jesuits, apart from Father

Coleridge and some of his close contemporaries, were even aware that Hopkins was a poet.

Still less, of course, was the Church, or Victorian society at large, aware of the fact, nor did Hopkins ever go out of his way to advertise his poetic wares. Even Bridges, who kept all the poems he had received, not without his own criticism, from his friend, judged that the time wasn't ripe for publication till thirty years had elapsed since his death in 1889. Why then blame the Society of Jesus or the Catholic Church for not having recognized the value of poems that White himself seems unwilling to recognize?

Turning now from the Catholic Church and the Society of Jesus in general to the deleterious influence they are imagined to have exerted on the poetry of Hopkins, White continually presents this in terms of an awkward transition he discerns in the poems from the delicate description of the natural world in the octave, which is for him the characteristic response of the poet, to the supervening imposition of a narrow moralistic dogma, which is for him the characteristic reflection of the priest. This transition is what White repeatedly returns to in the instance not of any Dublin poem but of the earlier sonnet on "Spring", which is ever preying on his mind.

Thus he laments the way "the sestet starts with a startling (sic) contrast: 'What is all this juice and all this joy?'"; and he goes on to assume that for Hopkins "all nature is a fable, and that as a priest he has the key and is the intermediary and interpreter". This is what he subsequently calls "a jerky change of voice", "an awkward change of attention halfway through", and a "shrill confidence in an over-wide viewpoint". Or again, it is what White sees as an attempt to force natural perception "within the limits of the narrow dogma he is expounding", as the poet's native freedom is "taken over by the simplistically limited but all-powerful forces of orthodoxy". Or yet again, it is what he calls "a clumsy standing back from the octave's subject matter".

After all, what White admires in this sonnet is all too narrowly restricted to the first eight lines of natural description, which is for him the only constituent of true poetry. And so, he continues, "the octave is too powerful to play merely a subordinate role to the moralistic sestet, and drowns the fable in 'juice and joy'." How astonished he might have been to hear the poet's voice from beyond the grave, if in the words of T. S. Eliot: "That is not it at all, That is not what I meant at all."

When he comes to the Dublin poems, this is again what White objects to, as, for example, in "Carrion Comfort" (where he wrongly glosses "carrion" as "both flesh and non-flesh", and "comfort" as "encouragement"). He lambastes the poem as "a conflation of disparate elements into a sonnet form which confers a superficial unity at odds with the material"—a material which for him lacks the natural perception of the earlier, brighter poems. In it he still admits a powerful description of despair; but he objects to Hopkins's way of "introducing traditional images" into the description so as to break up "the poem's continuity".

In general, White observes, "Conformity to the correct ideological stance destroys genuine continuity", and so he takes the poet to task for having derived his answers "from the Bible, not from reality"—as if "reality", in his sense of the word, has any answers to give. He further divides the poem into four sections, which he sees as "quite distinct, with artificial hinges, betraying their discontinuity". Again, he finds "there is naivety and superficiality in this quick application of emasculated metaphor to substantial troubles"—though again we might ask where is the superficiality, on the side of the poet or of his critic?

As for the last line, with its awed realization that the poet has, like Jacob, been wrestling with God himself, White can discern no sense of humble awe, but only "the pride that comes with the Jacob-like realization . . . that his wrestling adversary was no less than God", and "the self-congratulatory tone" that "leaves the poem in pieces"—in short, nothing but "a demonstration of the clash between the priest and the poet".

Such—without going into more examples, which would only build up a sense of reiterated tedium—is the burden of White's relentless condemnation of the priest behind the poet in Hopkins. For White the priest, as official representative of a narrowly dogmatic and authoritarian Church and of a rigid, uncomprehending, unappreciative religious order, is altogether opposed to the natural, spontaneous emotions of the poet. The former is the Censor or Super-Ego, imposing its rigid structures of authority on the would-be inspiration of the latter's Libido. It is this contradictory juxtaposition of these two aspects or influences which is seen as running through all Hopkins's poems and radically undermining them, till there is hardly a poem, at all events none of those on which there is any lengthy comment in this book, which White can wholeheartedly commend.

Nor can the author see any good in this "clash" of opposing forces or tendencies, or what Hopkins himself recognized as a creative strain (as in Part I of "The Wreck"); but he would have the poet without the priest, the artist without the bonds of morality or religion, or in other words, a poet and artist of his own devising, such as Hopkins might have become if only he hadn't been received into the Catholic Church or admitted into the Society of Jesus.

White, it seems, has no patience with the poet of the mature poems from "The Wreck" onwards, whether in the bright or the dark period, for in them all the poet is excessively subsumed by the priest. Thus, in the literal sense of the word, he is a rank "heretic" in his understanding of Hopkins, not only in differing from the Hopkinsian "orthodoxy", but also in picking and choosing those bits and pieces among the poems which catch his fancy (which is what the Greek word "heretic" originally means). He cannot take the poems as they are or make sense of them as a whole, but he is always imposing his personal prejudices on them, his own ideas as to how the poems ought to have been composed to suit his post-modern, post-Christian sensitivity.

In conclusion, after a careful perusal of this book, I am left with a feeling similar to that of Othello concerning poor Desdemona: "But yet the pity of it, Iago! O, Iago, the pity of it, Iago!" This is, however, no longer the simple pity I have expressed at the beginning of this article. Rather, within it I can analyse three separate feelings as brought together by White's book. First, there is White's own feeling of pity for a poet whose natural inspiration has been undermined, "distorted and sabotaged" (as he puts it) by "the moral straitjacket" imposed by his Church and his Society. Secondly, there is my own feeling of pity for White's inability to appreciate the total inspiration of Hopkins, arising as it does not just from a perception of the natural world, but from a creative tension between the priest and the poet. As I read Hopkins's poems, the priest in them isn't merely exercising a stern veto, or presiding over them with such a power always up his sleeve, but he is rather pointing to a heavenly source of light and energy beyond White's understanding.

Finally, I have a further feeling of pity for the way Hopkins is so unjustly and unmercifully criticized by White, who professes to know little, without seeking to know anything more, about the reality of either the Catholic Church or the Society of Jesus; but he remains content to look on his chosen subject, like Othello looking on Desdemona, with the jaundiced eyes of prejudice.

(*Hopkins Research* 33, December 2004)

Main Index

Adoro Te Devote (St. Thomas), 182
advice, 27, 29, 41, 50, 181, 186
"Age and Death" (Blake), 17
alliterative, alliteration, 20, 69, 121, 125, 191, 192, 199
alternation, 46
America, 62, 63, 120, 156
Anglicanism, 89, 90, 93, 94, 96, 120, 145, 147, 149, 180, 181, 187
annunciation, 158
anti-Catholic, 120
Apologia pro Vita Sua (Newman), 90–95, 122, 147, 164, 169, 176, 180, 181
Aquinas, St. Thomas, 111, 134, 169, 182, 201, 202
Arnold, Matthew, 91, 95
art, 5, 75, 77, 79, 190, 192, 199
As You Like It (Shakespeare), 177
"Ash Wednesday" (Eliot), 120

assonance, 20, 121, 125
bad taste, 93
Balliol College, 58, 59, 93, 180, 189
beauty, 2, 5–7, 10, 11, 13, 19, 28, 29, 34–36, 52, 66–68, 76, 102, 111, 112, 116, 125, 132, 133, 136, 151, 168, 173, 176, 192, 194, 200
Benarth, 10
Bergonzi, Bernard, 148
Birmingham Oratory, 92, 94, 95, 97, 147, 164, 180, 183, 190
Bischoff, Fr. Anthony, 57
Blake, William, 16–18
Blessed Virgin, 63, 70, 71, 111, 116, 157, 158
Bliss, Fr. Geoffrey, 56
Bond, Edward, 148
Bridges, Robert, 10, 11, 38, 39, 51, 74, 77, 96, 99, 100–103, 129, 147, 160, 165, 184, 189, 192, 194–96, 202

bright, 5, 9, 26, 36, 50–52, 69, 107, 108, 112–14, 124, 127, 136, 152, 159, 160, 173, 181, 182, 206
Browning, Robert, 53, 70, 77, 161
Byron, Lord George Gordon, 78, 192
Cantwell, Laurence, 59
Caroline, 89
Catholic, 18, 30, 41, 46, 66, 71, 74, 78, 89–95, 120, 145, 147, 148, 163, 164, 169, 174, 180, 181, 190, 197, 198, 200, 201, 203, 205, 207
chant, 38, 202
Charbeneau, Tom, 60
Church of England (see Anglicanism)
circling, 65–67, 69, 94, 97
Clark, Francis, 59
Clwyd, 9, 10
Coleridge, Fr. Henry, 202, 203
Coleridge, Samuel Taylor, 100, 180
Commentary on G. M. Hopkins' The Wreck of the Deutschland, A (Milward), 61
Commentary on the Sonnets of G. M. Hopkins, A (Milward), 61
"Commonitorium" (St. Vincent of Lerins), 91
Confessions (St. Augustine), 171

"Contemplation in Action" (Conwell), 172
conversion, 13, 66, 82, 83, 85, 92, 93, 95, 97, 120, 123, 126, 145, 147, 150, 157, 164, 167, 181, 184, 186, 190
Conwell, Fr. Joseph, 172, 173
Cowper, William, 108
Dante, 103
dapple, 2, 6, 111, 114, 125
Descartes, René, 187
Deutschland, the, 58, 81, 145, 156, 164, 169
development, 91, 92, 127, 164, 179
"Ding, dong, bell", 121
disyllables, 38
Divina Commedia (Dante), 103
Dixon, Canon, 15–19, 38, 51, 73–78, 100, 119, 148, 150, 153
Don Juan (Byron), 192
Donne, John, 191
dove, 36, 65, 66, 69–71, 181
"Dover Beach" (Arnold), 95
Dragon at the Gate, The (Schneider), 15, 101
Dryden, John, 23
Dublin, 31, 36, 51, 62, 74, 77, 92, 97, 107, 127, 128, 138, 146, 148, 154, 179, 183, 184, 186, 197, 198, 203, 204
ecceitas, 33, 112
eccentricity, 54, 56, 168, 189–96

Index of Poems Cited

echo, 1, 19–23, 29, 34, 35, 39, 52, 53, 61, 69, 70, 81, 94–96, 107, 112, 115, 119, 122, 132, 133, 138–42, 146, 147, 150–52, 160, 165–67, 185
ecology, 105
Eliot, T. S., 18, 20, 73, 120, 137, 145, 154, 200, 204
Elwy, 9–13, 69, 100–102, 135, 152
English Literary Society of Japan, 61
Enozawa, Kazuyoshi, 61
Essay on the Development of Christian Doctrine (Newman), 91, 92, 164
Faber, Frederick William, 148
Farm Street, 55, 183
favoured symbol, 65
Fichte, Johann Gottlieb, 187
Froude, Hurrell, 90
Genesareth, 16, 84, 124
Gerard Manley Hopkins (Bergonzi), 148
Gerard Manley Hopkins and the Victorian Temper (Sulloway), 15
"Gerontion" (Eliot), 18
Glasnevin, 62, 198
Grammar of Assent (Newman), 148, 154, 163–69
grammar, 45–47, 121, 191
Gray, Thomas, 50
Great Tradition, The (Leavis), 73

great poems, 95, 120, 129, 161, 164
haecceitas, 6, 33, 112–14
half-way house, 94, 96, 97, 145, 147, 180
Hamada, 60
Hamlet (Shakespeare), 137–43
Harriott, John, 59
Harris, Daniel A., 44–48
heart, 1, 2, 9, 13, 18, 27, 30, 31, 34, 40, 41, 50, 53, 56, 66, 67, 68, 81, 82, 87, 90, 96, 97, 100, 101–103, 109, 113, 114, 123, 125, 127, 132–36, 138, 140, 149, 150, 153, 154, 156, 158, 159, 166, 167, 171, 179, 181, 184–86, 193, 200
heretic, 44, 206
Hiroshima, 60
Hokuseido Press, 61
"Home Thoughts from Abroad" (Browning), 70
Hopkins, Gerard Manley
LIFE
1866, received into the Church by Newman, 93, 94, 95, 147
1868, enters religious life, 31, 95, 119, 120, 155, 181, 182, 197
1889, dies, 96, 128, 203
WORKS
See separate index
Hopkins in Ireland (White), 198

Hopkins Society, 61, 62
Immaculate Conception, 111, 116, 157
immaculate conception, 156
"In Memoriam" (Tennyson), 95
inferior poem, 58
Inferno (Dante), 103
inscape, 9, 13, 50, 63, 121–25, 125, 149, 176, 190
Inspirations Unbidden (Harris), 44
instress, 13, 35, 121, 122, 125, 149, 190
"Intimations of Immortality" (Wordsworth), 75, 150
Ireland, 139, 148, 198, 200
Japan, 55, 56, 59, 61–63, 129
Kant, Immanuel, 46, 187
Keats, John, 73–76, 78, 100
Keble, John, 90, 148
King Lear (Shakespeare), 61, 140, 143
Kingsley, Charles, 92
Korea, 62
Lake Kawaguchi, 59
Lancashire, 11, 176
Landscape and Inscape (Milward), 63
Langland, William, 191
"Lead, kindly Light" (Newman), 90, 95, 146, 147, 153
Leavis, F. R., 73
Letter to the Hebrews, 27
liberal, 89, 90, 94

Liddon, Henry, 93, 180
Liverpool, 38, 39, 183
Lombard, Peter, 111
Loyola, 62, 80
"Lycidas" (Milton), 76
Maenefa, 10, 151
marriage, 156, 160
Measure for Measure (Shakespeare), 140, 176
method, 20, 85, 168
Miller, Alfred, 100
Milton, John, 74, 76–78, 100, 112, 121, 129, 192, 194–96
monosyllables, 38, 124, 125,
Month, The, 121, 191, 202
moral, 17, 31, 79, 80, 82, 86, 185, 192, 199, 200, 203, 204–206
More, Sir Thomas, 157
Mount Fuji, 59, 60
Nadal, Fr. Jerome, 172, 173
"National Apostasy, The" (Keble), 90
Neri, St. Philip, 92
Newman, John Henry, 1, 71, 89–97, 122, 123, 127, 146–50, 153, 154, 163–69, 176, 180, 181, 183, 187, 190
North British Review, 149
North Sea, 16, 124, 145
odd, 12, 56, 193, 194, 196
Okumura, Prof. Mifune, 61
Oratory, 92, 94, 95, 147, 164, 168, 183
Oriel College, 90, 92

Index of Poems Cited

Oxford Movement, 17, 89, 92, 93, 95, 164, 180
Paradise Lost (Milton), 112, 192
Paradiso (Dante), 103
parallelism, 45, 47
Parmenides, 121, 149, 190
parson, 30
Patmore, Coventry, 74, 148, 155
Penseés (Pascal), 166
Phoenix and the Turtle (Shakespeare), 166
pied, 2, 6, 66, 111, 116, 132, 168, 192
Pierce Ploughman, 191
Piers Plowman (Langland), 121
"Pillar of Cloud, The" (Newman), 146
Pindar, 76, 80, 165, 190
Poets and the Poetry of the Century, The (Miller), 100
Poets' Corner, 63
Prelude, The (Wordsworth), 26, 149
procreation, 155, 158, 160
Protestantism, 30, 89, 91, 124, 202
Purcell, Henry, 23, 34, 77
Purgatorio (Dante), 103
Pusey, Edward Bouverie, 92, 93, 180
"Rabbi Ben Ezra" (Browning), 53, 77
renunciation, 3, 31, 35, 36, 101, 103

Rhyl, 10, 12, 106
rhythm, 2, 38, 46, 76, 77, 119, 121–27, 190, 191
Ribble, 11, 106, 108, 135, 176, 182, 193
Richard II (Shakespeare), 194
Roman Church, 89, 91, 94, 145
Royal University, 127
Ruskin, John, 108, 190
Russell, Lord John, 89
sacrifice, 27, 29, 31, 32, 35, 36, 133, 134, 136, 147, 168
Samson Agonistes (Milton), 77, 121
Schneider, Elisabeth, 15, 16
Schoder, Fr. Raymond, 58, 60, 62–64
"Scotus on the Sentences" (Scotus), 34, 38, 57, 59, 106, 111–13, 116, 169, 188, 192, 193, 201
Seoul, 62
Shairp, J. C., 149
Shakespeare, William, 47, 54, 61, 73–78, 84, 100, 108, 137–39, 142, 143, 166, 167, 175, 177, 179, 182, 188, 191, 194, 195
Shelley, Percy Bysshe, 53, 67, 73, 100, 105, 107, 161
Shimane Prefecture, 60
Sogang University, 62
"Song for St. Cecilia's Day" (Dryden), 23
Sophia University, 60, 62

Spirit of Man, The (Bridges), 40, 99, 102, 103
Spiritual Exercises (St. Ignatius), 68, 82, 126, 168, 180
St. Anselm, 187
St. Asaph, 10
St. Augustine, 89, 171
St. Beuno's College, 9, 10, 13, 36, 55, 56, 58, 62, 63, 65, 68, 80, 105, 119, 124, 127, 145, 151, 181, 183, 190, 198, 202
St. Francis Xavier's Church, 38, 39, 183
St. Ignatius, 68, 80, 81, 82, 92, 126, 168, 171–73, 175, 177, 180, 181, 187, 192
St. John of the Cross, 127
St. Mary (see Blessed Virgin)
St. Mary's, 55, 57, 90, 91, 111, 165, 183
St. Peter, 17, 18, 94
St. Teresa of Avila, 176, 185
St. Vincent of Lerins, 91
Stonyhurst, 55, 57, 62, 111–13, 165, 169, 176, 183
Suarez, 169
Sulloway, Alison, 15–17
symmetry, 5
syntax, 38, 191
Taura (Japan), 59

Tempest, The (Shakespeare), 182
Tennyson, Lord Alfred, 74, 75, 78, 95
terrible, 3, 55, 56, 61, 96, 127, 197
Teutonic, 38
Thirty-nine Articles, the, 90
touchiness, 163
Tractarianism, 90–92, 164
"Tradition and the Individual Talent" (Eliot), 73
"Tyger, The" (Blake), 17, 18
underthought, 61, 137, 140
Urquhart, Edward, 149
Utopia (More), 157
Veni Creator Spiritus, 155, 175
verbum, 39, 134
Via Media, 90
vocation, 25, 26, 41, 66, 80, 120, 200
Wales, 9–13, 119, 145, 198
Westminster Abbey, 63
Whig, 89
White, Norman, 198–206
Whitman, Walt, 20
Wilberforce, William, 17
Wordsworth, William, 15–17, 26, 27, 75–78, 100, 149–54, 165, 179, 194
Yeats, W. B., 157

Index of Poems Cited

Alchemist in the City, 65, 200
Andromeda, 36, 77, 139, 195–96
As kingfishers catch fire, 21, 116, 168, 192–93
At the Wedding March, 132
Binsey Poplars, 33, 34, 132, 139, 142, 176, 182
Blessed Virgin compared to the Air, The, 70, 116
Bugler's First Communion, The, 30, 35, 167–68
Caged Skylark, The, 68–69, 133
Candle Indoors, The, 34, 100–102, 182
Carrion Comfort, 16, 44, 51, 96, 114, 115, 140, 142, 143, 165, 204
Felix Randal, 30, 132, 135, 142, 183
God's Grandeur, 51, 69, 105–107, 113, 114, 131, 136, 152, 159, 173, 174, 182, 183
Habit of Perfection, The, 100, 101, 103

Half-way House, The, 94–97, 145, 147, 180
Handsome Heart, The, 34, 35, 66, 100, 101, 103, 132
Henry Purcell, 23, 34, 138, 202
Hurrahing in Harvest, 10, 13, 27, 51, 66, 112, 159
In the Valley of the Elwy, 9–12, 13, 69, 100, 101, 102, 103, 135, 152
Inversnaid, 20–22, 51, 62, 152
I wake and feel, 43–48, 115, 169, 179
Lantern Out of Doors, The, 34, 138
Leaden Echo and the Golden Echo, The, 19–22, 29, 35, 132–33
Let me be to Thee, 65, 69, 94, 97
Loss of the Eurydice, The, 22, 28, 97, 139–40, 194–96, 202
May Magnificat, The, 69, 70, 113, 116, 152, 159

Moonrise, 151
Morning, Midday, and Evening Sacrifice, The, 29, 35, 133
My own heart, 127, 179, 185
Myself unholy, 65
Nondum, 94, 96, 146
Nightingale, The, 65
No worst, there is none, 47, 140
Patience, 36, 115, 135, 169
Peace, 36, 70
Penmaen Pool, 58
Pied Beauty, 6, 7, 111, 116, 132, 168, 192
Ribblesdale, 106, 108, 135, 176, 182, 193
S. Thomae Aquinatis Rhythmus, 72
St. Winefred's Well, 19, 55, 78
Sea and the Skylark, The, 12, 106
Shepherd's Brow, The, 76
Soldier, The, 114
Spelt from Sibyl's Leaves, 6, 7, 50–52, 77, 114, 139, 141, 199, 201
Spring, 28, 29, 69, 70, 131, 152, 153, 159, 203
Spring and Fall, 37, 38, 40, 41, 100–102, 152, 167, 195

Starlight Night, The, 112, 151
That Nature is a Heraclitean Fire, 48–51, 60, 77, 96, 115, 128, 135, 143, 153, 161, 186
Thou art indeed just, Lord, 160, 199
To what serves Mortal Beauty?, 29, 35, 132, 136, 168
To seem the stranger, 47, 138, 141, 160, 169, 179, 197
To R. B., 53, 115, 160
Vision of Mermaids, A, 74
Windhover, The, 1, 2, 3, 61, 62, 67, 68, 114, 124–26, 151, 158, 200
Wreck of the Deutschland, The, 1, 3, 9, 12, 15, 16, 17, 21, 22, 25, 28, 37–40, 48, 51–53, 56, 60, 61, 66, 69, 76, 77, 80–82, 87, 95–97, 100–102, 112, 113, 119, 120, 121, 123–29, 133–41, 145, 146, 148, 150–53, 156, 158–60, 164–68, 174, 175, 181, 182, 190–92, 194, 202, 205

DUE DATE

FEB 24 1991				
AUG 12 1991				
DEC 27				
MAY 09 1996				
MAY 13 1997				

A Root

F
HED
#7062

Hedberg, Nancy.
A rooted sorrow.

$6.95

DATE DUE	BORROWER'S NAME	ROOM NUMBER
FEB 24 199	Helen ...	

F
HED
#7062

Hedberg, Nancy.
A rooted sorrow.

$6.95

CHRIST UNITED METHODIST CHURCH
4488 POPLAR AVENUE
MEMPHIS, TENNESSEE 38117